Spiralizer Cookbook

Simple, Delicious and Healthy Spiralizer Recipes Made for Everyone

Table of Contents

Introduction

It might not seem all that impressive, but that little Spiralizer sitting on your counter is one of the most useful tools in your kitchen. So, if you've ever looked at it and wondered if it was worth it? Well, the short answer is yes! Your Spiralizer does so much more than turn zucchinis into noodles. Now, if you just purchased it for that reason I really don't blame you, zucchini noodles are great. But you should know that if you're *only* making zoodles, then you're definitely missing out. And who likes to miss out on delicious food? No one!

That's why I created my cookbook *Simple, Delicious and Healthy Spiralizer Recipes Made for Everyone* so I could share plenty of delicious recipes made with different kinds of vegetable and fruit noodles. With my cookbook, you'll be able to make everything from nutritious salads to tasty appetizers, filling entrees, and even healthy desserts! I'll also be sharing with you all the benefits of owning a spiralizer, along with helpful tips so you can use it like a pro.

Now, let's get into how your amazing spiralizer works and why it's so great below!

The Spiralizer - What is it?

Everyone from home to restaurant chefs are spiralizing veggies. Why? To make fresh faux-noodles of course. But what exactly is a spiralizer and how does it turn your favorite vegetables into tasty spiralized ribbons?

In short, a spiralizer is a kitchen tool that pretty much works like a giant pencil sharpener. Just place a firm, peeled vegetable in place with a clamp over the grinder/blade, then you just use the hand crank to turn the gears. The end result will be extra-long, semi-curled vegetable ribbons or noodles. And that's it! Just spin and trim, and you'll have a bowl full of vegetable noodles to create whatever you want.

Now, besides being extra easy to use, your spiralizer offers a lot of benefits to almost every aspect of your life. And that's exactly what we'll be getting into next.

The Benefits of Owning a Spiralizer

From your overall health to saving time, your spiralizer has plenty of benefits that will transform your life! You're probably wondering what they are, right? Below you'll find 10 unique benefits that will motivate you to spiralize whenever you can.

Healthy Weight Loss, Detox and Maintenance

When you opt to spiralize all your veggies, you'll naturally eat more vegetables without even noticing it – especially when you top it with a delicious sauce. This higher intake of fresh vegetables and high-quality fiber means you'll be able to optimize your energy levels and stay satisfied for much longer. Just this tiny shift in your eating habits will lead to weight loss since you're consuming more vegetables and less processed foods.

Most veggies are really rich in water - for example, vegetables like cucumbers are made up of 95% water - along with tons of antioxidants that help with tissue detoxification. While hydrating vegetables like zucchinis will help your body flush out even more toxins. Plus, other vegetables like broccoli can even help kick-start your metabolism. So, after you eat a bowl of vegetable noodles, you'll feel much lighter and more energized!

Improve Your Diet and Meal Preferences

Whether you're on a low-carb diet, vegetable-based diet, paleo diet, or weight loss diet, a spiralizer is an excellent way to improve the taste, look and aroma of your meals. Spiralized vegetables and fruits are also super helpful for people who have an autoimmune disease, like Celiac and those with food sensitivities to gluten. Vegetables are a top choice to replace rice, regular pasta, and noodles that are mainly made out of rice, wheat or flour since spiralized vegetables are totally clean and unprocessed.

Makes the Most Out of Your Vegetables and Fruits

When you use a knife to chop, dice or cube vegetables – you barely get a cupful. On the other hand, when you have a spiralizer one small vegetable can give many cups of fluffy, spiral vegetables. This means that those vegetables and fruits can go a very long way. You'll also end up feeling like you're eating a really big portion, when in fact it's a moderate amount of spiralized vegetables. For example, one medium red potato spiralized will be enough for two people to share.

Sneak More Vegetables into Your Diet Without Sacrificing Flavor

Spiralized vegetables have such a similar texture and consistency to regular Italian noodles and pasta, that your taste buds won't even know the difference! So, once you can start replacing the carbs with vegetables and fruits, slowly but surely, you'll be adding way more vegetables into your overall diet.

Encourages You to Eat Locally and Seasonally, and Reduces Your Carbon Footprint

With a Spiralizer in your kitchen, you're more likely to head to the farmer's market to search for fresh produce in different shapes and sizes. And by shopping at the farmers market, you'll support your local farm community, reduce your carbon footprint, and you'll naturally start to eat seasonally!

A lot of vegetables (including zucchinis) get smaller in size during the off-season, which makes them more difficult to spiralize. So, while you're out and about strolling to each vegetable stand you're bound to discover new seasonal vegetables and become even more creative in the kitchen, all while being eco-friendly.

Effortlessly Make More Kid-Friendly and Family-Friendly Meals

If you have kids, they will love watching a vegetable or fruit instantly turn into noodles right before their eyes. And as long as they're supervised, the kiddos can help in the spiralizing process too! When you do this together, your children will learn about healthy habits while having fun. Plus, they'll be more willing to eat those magically made veggie or fruit noodles.

Spiralizing is also the quickest way to prepare a lot of vegetables at one time, so it's definitely family-friendly! For example, you won't have to wait around for water to boil to cook pasta noodles. You can just spiralize a few vegetables and cook it in just a few minutes. This way you can spend less time in the kitchen and more time with your family.

You'll Get More Creative in the Kitchen

It's no secret that spiralizing your veggies and fruits will really challenge you to come up with some new creative meals with all the noodles you've made. And since each vegetable and fruit have their own flavors, textures, and nutrients, things can get very interesting. You can always opt to invent your own inspirational meal by adding the noodles to whatever dish you'd like or reinvent a classic with your veggie noodles - think omelet with spiralized peppers or lasagna with spiralized zucchini.

One thing's for sure, you'll never get bored with a spiralizer and you'll definitely look forward to making something new each time!

Spiralizing Makes Vegetables and Fruit Cook Faster

Finally, stop wasting time standing in the kitchen prepping vegetables and fruits by slicing and dicing them all up. With a spiralizer in your kitchen, it will take just seconds to prep ready-to-cook noodles, and just a couple of minutes to actually cook them. Plus, this also means no more boiling water, starchy pasta water or mushy rice!

Keep the Nutrition Value

Did you know that if you cook your vegetables at the wrong temperature or overcook them you can actually destroy their nutritional value? Nutrients such as vitamins, antioxidants, minerals, and proteins happen to be very sensitive to high temperatures.

So, when you prepare vegetables the traditional way by cutting them into cubes or thick slices, you can easily overcook them or cook them at a high temperature for too long and lower their nutritional value. But when you spiralize you're fruits and veggies into to uniform noodles, you're able to avoid cooking them for way too long or overheating them.

Anyone Can Use a Spiralizer

Whether you're an at-home mom, college student or a hard-working individual, a vegetable spiralizer will give you the opportunity to cook delicious, healthy meals without having tons of prior cooking experience! Dinnertime will become much easier, healthier and a whole lot faster.

Spiralizer Tips

My cookbook wouldn't be complete without a few tips that will help you use your Spiralizer like a pro! Now let's jump into my top 8 tips for spiralizing.

Try Out All the Blades

Don't be afraid to play around with the different blades you have. You might want to have your slices thicker or thinner depending on the vegetable or recipe.

Watch out For Brightly Colored Vegetables

Vegetables that are orange and red/purple colored are packed with nutrients since they get their color from beta-carotene and anthocyanin – but these bright colors can also stain your Spiralizer. So, remember to immediately wash the spiralizer (and cutting board) after spiralizing any kind of brightly colored veggies.

Look for Wide Vegetables

When you spiralize vegetables like carrots, parsnips, and others that are "narrow", grab the largest ones you can find. With a Spiralizer, the wider the vegetable the better.

Make Meal Prep Easier

Many spiralized vegetables are great for meal prep. You can slice the zucchini, carrot, onion, and beets on the weekend and store in a ziploc bag or container in the fridge and use throughout the week.

Trim Your Noodles

If you could continuously spiralize a vegetable, you'll end up with one extremely long noodle and even cause the blade to jam. Keep this from happening by slicing the noodle while spiralizing. It also helps with serving since you'll end up with regular-sized noodles that you can divide and eat.

Here's How You Can Make Your Sauce Less Watery

When you're cooking vegetables, keep in mind that your sauce can get a bit watery. So the longer the noodles stay the sauce, the more watery it will be. To prevent this you can also cook the noodles ahead of time in a separate skillet. Then take the noodles out with a slotted spoon, pat dry with paper towels and set aside for when you're ready to add them to the sauce.

Enjoy the Veggie Noodles Raw
Instead of cooking the noodles, skip that step and add the raw crunchy noodles to a plate or bowl and simply pour a warm sauce on top. The noodles will slightly heat up and soften.

Avoid Making Half-Moon Noodles
To avoid the spiralizer slicing the vegetables into half-moons, make sure the vegetable isn't moving off the center by repositioning it back in place when needed. You can also flip the vegetables around. If you do end up with a pile of half-moons, don't throw them out! Use them to make a fresh pasta salad with your favorite dressing.

Conclusion

After reading the benefits and pro tips you should be more than ready to get into the kitchen and start spiralizing your favorite vegetables and fruits. Like I mentioned before, your creative inner chef will also start to show when you cook with the veggie or fruit noodles you've created.

But on those days when you need some inspiration or a lot of help, feel free to open my cookbook to create a variety of delicious recipes. You can make a spiralized meal 3 times a day if you'd like. And trust me, your taste buds, along with your family and friends will love these surprisingly healthy dishes too!

Each section in my cookbook features recipes that anyone can make (so, if you can turn on an oven, you can cook these recipes) and there's a variety of choices in each section too!

Your morning wouldn't be complete without breakfast, so be sure to flip to the **Breakfast** section to find both sweet and savory recipes that feature fruit and vegetable noodles. There's everything from zucchini banana bread to spiralized apple oatmeal bowls and classic veggie omelets.

When it's time to throw a party, don't go out and buy store-bought appetizers! Instead, whip up everything you need in your own kitchen. Just flip to the **Appetizer** section for crowd-pleasing recipes to create mini snacks like crispy veggie fritters, spiral home fries, spring rolls and much more.

Easily make a flavorful meal for the whole family with the recipes in my **Seafood**, **Beef** and **Chicken** section. In these sections, you'll find a variety of recipes so you can create marinated beef, grilled fish, and crispy Parmesan chicken served with veggie noodles.

On those days when you want something light and healthy, check out my **Vegetarian and Vegan** section. The recipes here will turn your vegetable noodles into delicious, filling meals such as zucchini stir-fry, yellow squash pasta, and loaded veggie salad.

When you want to indulge in something sweet, my **Dessert** section is ready for you to enjoy! You can turn apples, pears and peaches into yummy (and pretty healthy) dessert bars, yogurt parfaits, and muffins.

Now, what are you waiting for? It's time to set up your spiralizer and start cooking!

Recipes

Breakfast

Breakfast Butternut Squash Risotto with Bacon and Fried Egg

You won't be able to get enough of this breakfast risotto! Made with butternut squash "risotto", bacon and a fried egg, this savory dish is one filling breakfast.

Prep Time: 20 Minutes
Cook Time: 25 Minutes
Total Time: 45 Minutes
Yields 4

Ingredients:

Risotto:

- 1 large butternut squash, peeled, spiralized
- 1 Tbsp. olive oil
- 2 cloves of garlic, minced
- ½ cup chicken broth, more if needed
- ¼ cup shredded mild cheddar cheese
- ¼ cup shredded Havarti cheese
- Salt, to taste
- Pepper, to taste

Toppings:

- 4 strips of bacon
- 4 whole large eggs
- 2 Tbsp. freshly minced parsley, for garnish

Directions:

1. In a food processor, pulse the butternut squash noodles until rice-like, then set aside
2. Place a large skillet over medium-high heat
3. Once heated, add in the bacon and cook until crispy, then transfer the bacon to paper towel-lined sheet and set aside
4. In a large pot over medium heat, add 1 Tbsp. olive oil
5. Once the oil is heated, add in the garlic and cook for 30 seconds or until fragrant
6. Add in the butternut squash rice, season with salt and pepper and stir, cook for 2 minutes to heat through, then add the broth

7. Lower heat to low to bring to a simmer, cook for 10-15 minutes or until broth fully reduces
8. Remove the pan from the heat and fold in the cheeses, stir until cheese has fully melted and then top with the bacon crumbles and stir to combine, once the risotto is almost done, set aside
9. Using the same skillet that was used to cook the bacon, wipe it down and place it over medium-high heat, once heated, add in the eggs, cook the eggs until whites are set
10. Spoon risotto into bowls and top with the fried egg and garnish with parsley
11. Enjoy!

Nutritional Facts Per Serving |Calories: 220 |Carbs: 8g |Total Fat: 15g |Protein: 12g

Chocolate Chip Sweet Potato Waffles

Infused with cinnamon and dark chocolate, these Sweet Potato Waffles are an amazing treat for breakfast!

Prep Time: 10 Minutes
Cook Time: 20 Minutes
Total Time: 30 Minutes
Serves 2

Ingredients:

- 1 large sweet potato, peeled, spiralized, trimmed
- 1 large egg, beaten
- 2 Tbsp. chopped dark chocolate
- Salt, to taste
- ½ tsp. cinnamon
- Cooking spray

Optional Toppings:

- Maple syrup
- Blueberries
- Pecans

Directions:

1. Preheat your Belgian waffle iron
2. Place a large skillet over medium heat, add in the olive oil
3. Once heated, add in the sweet potatoes noodles and season with salt and cinnamon, toss and cook for about 10 minutes or until noodles are cooked through (You can also cover the pan to cook more quickly)
4. Transfer the sweet potato noodles to a large mixing bowl, add in the egg and chocolate, toss to combine
5. Spray the preheated waffle iron with cooking spray and pack in the noodles carefully
6. Cook the waffle according to your iron's settings instructions
7. Once done, carefully remove the waffles and transfer them to the plates
8. Top with the maple syrup and any additional toppings of your choice

Nutritional Facts Per Serving |Calories: 158 |Carbs: 23 g |Total Fat:6 g |Protein:5 g

Parsnip Noodle Nest topped with Eggs, Bacon and Arugula

Perfect for breakfast or brunch, this recipe delivers breakfast classics (bacon and eggs) on top of a crunchy spiralized parsnip noodle nest.

Prep Time: 5 Minutes
Cook Time: 40 Minutes
Total Time: 45 Minutes
Yields 8

Ingredients:

- 2 large parsnips, peeled, spiralized, trimmed
- 2 strips of bacon
- 1 cup baby arugula
- 2 eggs, beaten
- 8 whole eggs
- ½ tsp. garlic powder
- Salt, to taste
- Pepper, to taste
- Hot sauce, to drizzle
- Large muffin tin

Directions:

1. Preheat the oven to 425 degrees F
2. Grease a large muffin tin with the cooking spray
3. Place a large skillet over medium-high heat
4. Once heated, add in the bacon, cook for about 10 minutes, until cooked through and crispy, then set aside on a paper towel-lined plate
5. When the bacon has cooled, crumble into small bite size pieces
6. Remove all of the bacon fat except for about one Tbsp. and add in the parsnip noodles. Season with salt, pepper and garlic powder and toss. Cook for 5-7 minutes or until cooked through and then transfer to a medium mixing bowl. Allow it to cool for 2 minutes.
7. Add the eggs to the bowl and toss thoroughly to combine
8. Pack the parsnip noodles into the muffin tins, trying your best to create a hole in the center, cook for 15 minutes
9. Remove the parsnip nests from the oven and crack an egg in each one
10. Place the tin back in the oven and bake for another 9 to 12 minutes or until the eggs set
11. Open the oven and check after 9 minutes, give the muffin pan a shake and if the egg whites aren't set, cook for another 2 minutes and then check again
12. Once done, remove from the oven and top with the arugula, bacon and hot sauce, more if desired and serve

Nutritional Facts Per Serving |Calories: 92 |Carbs: 7g |Total Fat: 5g |Protein: 6g

Sweet Potato Pancakes

As you already know, traditional deep-fried potato pancakes aren't exactly healthy. That's why you can easily replace them with this 5 ingredient Sweet Potato pancake recipe!

Prep Time: 10 Minutes
Cook Time: 20 Minutes
Total Time: 30 Minutes
Serves: 4

Ingredients:

- 1 large (11 oz. peeled) sweet potato, cut in half, peeled and spiralized
- ½ cup chopped scallions
- 2 large eggs, beaten
- 4 cloves crushed garlic
- 4 tsp. olive oil
- ½ tsp. kosher salt
- Fresh black pepper, to taste

Directions:

1. Prepare the sweet potato by cutting them in half and spiralizing them with the small noodle blade on the spiralizer, cut into small pieces, about 5 inches long
2. In a large bowl, add the sweet potatoes, scallions, eggs, garlic, salt and pepper, mix well to combine
3. Place a large nonstick skillet over medium-low heat
4. Once heated, add 1 tsp. of oil, swirl to cover the pan
5. Using a fork, place about 1/3 cup of the sweet potato mixture, and gently place it in the skillet lightly pressing down with the fork, about 4 can fit onto the skillet
6. Cook until golden brown on the bottom, about 3 minutes then flip with a spatula, use the spatula to press them down to flatten and cook until golden, about 3 more minutes
7. Repeat the previous steps with the rest of the mixture
8. Serve

Nutritional Facts Calories: 125 |Carbs: 11g |Total Fat: 7g |Protein: 4.5g

Savory Parsnip Chive Waffles

Crispy with a soft middle, just top these Savory Parsnip Chive Waffle with bacon and Greek yogurt for a completely yummy breakfast.

Prep Time: 10 Minutes
Cook Time: 15 Minutes
Total Time: 25 Minutes
Yields: 4-8 Waffles

Ingredients:

- 2 large parsnips, peeled, spiralized, trimmed
- 1 large egg, beaten
- 3 Tbsp. chopped chives
- ½ Tbsp. extra virgin olive oil
- ¼ tsp. garlic powder
- Salt, to taste
- Pepper, to taste

Optional Toppings:

- ¼ cup Greek yogurt
- 2 tsp. lemon juice
- Bacon or Maple bacon

Directions:

1. Preheat a Belgian waffle iron
2. In the meantime, place a large skillet over medium heat and add in the olive oil
3. Once heated, add in the spiralized parsnip noodles and season with garlic powder, salt and pepper, cover and cook for 5 minutes, or until the noodles are wilted and cooked through
4. Once cooked, add the noodles to a bowl with the egg and chives, toss to combine
5. Spray the waffle iron with cooking spray and then add in some of the parsnip mixture
6. Cook according to your waffle iron's settings and then remove carefully
7. While the waffles are cooking, in a bowl mix together the optional Greek Yogurt, lemon juice and season with pepper
8. Once the waffles are done, top with optional Greek yogurt or serve as is, with salty bacon or maple syrup

Nutritional Facts Per Serving |Calories: 192 |Carbs: 30g |Total Fat: 7g |Protein: 5g

Bacon and Cheese Frittata with Spiral Potatoes

Start your breakfast with this delicious bacon and cheese frittata recipe that features spiralized potatoes and chives!

Prep Time: 10 Minutes
Cook Time: 30 Minutes
Total Time: 40 Minutes
Yields: 5 Servings

Ingredients:

- 2 small Yukon Gold potatoes, peeled, spiralized
- 4 slices bacon
- 8 large eggs
- 1 Tbsp. chopped chives
- ½ heaping cup shredded cheddar cheese
- ¼ tsp. garlic powder
- Salt, to taste
- Pepper, to taste

Directions:

1. Preheat the oven to 425 degrees F
2. Place a medium skillet over medium-high heat
3. Once heated, add in the bacon and cook for 5 minutes, flip, and then cook for another 5 minutes or until crispy and cooked through, transfer to a paper towel-lined plate
4. Immediately add the potato noodles to the pan, season with garlic powder, salt, and pepper, then toss in the bacon grease and allow them to cook thoroughly, tossing occasionally for about 7 minutes
5. In the meantime, crumble the bacon
6. In a medium bowl, whisk together the eggs add in the crumbled bacon, chives, and cheddar cheese, stir to combine
7. Once the potato noodles are done cooking, spread them out evenly on the bottom of the skillet
8. Pour the egg mixture over the potatoes and swirl the pan until eggs cover the potatoes, cook until the eggs set on the bottom, 2 to 3 minutes
9. Transfer the skillet into the oven and bake for 10-12 minutes or until eggs are completely set
10. Once completed, remove from the oven and slice into four or eight slices
11. Serve immediately

Nutritional Facts Per Serving |Calories: 276 |Carbs: 14g |Total Fat: 16g |Protein: 20g

Linguine and Zoodle Pasta with Poached Egg and Asparagus

Pasta for breakfast? With this linguine and zoodle pasta tossed with parmesan cheese and topped with a poached egg and asparagus, why not?

Prep Time: 10 Minutes
Cook Time: 15 Minutes
Total Time: 25 Minutes
Yields: 4 Servings

Ingredients:

- 1 bunch of asparagus trimmed and cut into bite-sized pieces
- 2 cups of snap peas, ends trimmed
- 4 cloves garlic, minced
- Zest and juice from one lemon
- ½ cup freshly grated parmesan cheese
- 4 eggs or more, if desired

For a ½ zoodle ½ linguine version:

- 4 oz. linguine
- 2 medium zucchinis, spiralized, 8 loosely packed cups

Directions:

1. Cook the pasta according to directions on the package
2. In the meantime, heat a large pan or skillet over medium heat
3. Once heated, add the asparagus and snap peas, and cook for 3 minutes
4. Then add in the zucchini noodles and garlic, cook for 3 to 4 minutes, mixing frequently with tongs or a fork
5. Once the zucchini noodles are cooked, add the lemon zest, lemon juice and parmesan cheese
6. When the pasta is done, scoop out the noodles from the boiling water, don't drain yet and add to the pan with the zucchini, toss evenly and arrange on plates
7. Drain all the water except for 2 inches of water from the pasta pot
8. Then crack the eggs into the water, cook for 3 minutes, or until eggs are cooked to your liking, once cooked scoop them out of the water and place them on top of the pasta
9. Serve!

Nutritional Facts Per Serving (¼ batch) |Calories:235 |Carbs: 14g |Total Fat: 13g |Protein: 17g

Breakfast Omelets with Spiralized Bell Peppers

Make your breakfast omelet even more flavorful with fresh tomatoes along with peppers and onion noodles.

Prep Time: 10 Minutes
Cook Time: 10 Minutes
Total Time: 20 Minutes
Yields 1

Ingredients:

- 1 tsp. extra virgin olive oil
- 1 red or green bell pepper, spiralized, trimmed
- ½ small white or yellow onion, spiralized, trimmed
- 2 eggs, beaten
- 1/3 cup diced tomatoes
- ¼ avocado, pitted, peeled and sliced
- ¼ tsp. dried thyme
- Salt, to taste
- Pepper, to taste

To Serve:

- Green salad
- Salsa

Directions:

1. Place a 10" skillet over medium-high heat, add the olive oil
2. Spiralize the peppers and onion with a small blade
3. Once heated, add the bell peppers, onions and season with thyme, salt and pepper, cook until soft, about 5-7 minutes
4. Then pour in the beaten eggs, tilting the pan to allow the eggs to fill the bottom of the pan
5. Sprinkle with the diced tomatoes, cook for 2 minutes until eggs set on the bottom, then run a spatula around the edges and then under the omelet to loosen it from the pan and flip it over
6. Allow the omelet to cook for 2 more minutes and then fold in half, gently pressing down with the spatula
7. Transfer the cooked omelet to a plate and top with the avocado slices
8. Serve with the green salad and salsa, if desired

Nutritional Facts Per Serving |Calories: 327 |Carbs: 22g |Total Fat: 20g |Protein: 16g

Zucchini Banana Bread

Sweet and soft, this easy to make Zucchini Banana Bread is a satisfying and healthy choice for breakfast!

Prep Time: 15 Minutes
Cook Time: 40 Minutes
Total Time: 55 Minutes
Yields 1 Loaf

Ingredients:

- 3 eggs
- 1 ½ cups coconut flour
- 2 very ripe bananas, mashed
- 1 medium zucchini, spiralized with a med.size blade, trimmed
- 1 tsp. baking soda
- ¾ tsp. ground cinnamon
- ½ tsp. salt
- ¼ cup maple syrup
- 2 tsp. vanilla extract
- 2 Tbsp. coconut oil, melted and cooled to room temperature
- 2 Tbsp. almond milk and more if needed
- ¾ cup walnuts, chopped
- 1 banana, halved lengthwise

Directions:

1. Preheat the oven to 350 degrees F
2. Grease a bread loaf pan with cooking spray, set aside
3. In a medium bowl, add in the coconut flour, baking soda, cinnamon, and salt
4. In a separate medium bowl, mix together the banana, eggs, maple syrup, almond milk, vanilla extract and coconut oil
5. Add in the dry ingredients with the wet, stir well until smooth
6. Then add in the zucchini and stir to combine, then fold in the walnuts and stir again
7. Pour the batter into the loaf pan and place the banana halves down into the batter, pressing slightly. Bake for 40 minutes or until a toothpick comes out clean from the center
8. Remove the loaf from the oven
9. Allow the bread loaf to cool for 5 minutes before slicing
10. Enjoy!

Nutritional Facts Per Serving without walnuts| Calories: 207 |Carbs: 26g |Total Fat: 8g |Protein: 6g

Nutritional Facts Per Serving with walnuts| Calories: 282|Carbs: 28g |Total Fat: 16g |Protein: 8g

Pumpkin Spice Sweet Potato Waffles

Brighten up your morning with the smell of these aromatic Pumpkin Spice Sweet Potato Waffles!

Prep Time: 5 Minutes
Cook Time: 20 Minutes
Total Time: 25 Minutes
Yields: 1-2 Servings

Ingredients:

- 1 medium sweet potato, peeled, spiralized
- 1 tsp. pumpkin spice
- 1 medium egg, beaten
- 1 Tbsp. maple syrup or more, to preference
- Cooking spray

Directions:

1. Preheat the waffle iron
2. Spiralize the sweet potato with a small blade, trim and set aside
3. Place a large skillet over medium heat, coat with the cooking spray
4. Once heated, add in the sweet potato noodles, cook turning frequently, for about 10 minutes or until the noodles have softened
5. Add the noodles into a bowl season with the pumpkin spice, mix to combine thoroughly
6. Add in the beaten egg, toss to combine
7. Spray the waffle iron with cooking spray and pack in the noodles, making sure they fit into all the grooves
8. Cook the waffle according to your iron's settings
9. Once cooked, serve with maple syrup

Nutritional Facts Per Serving |Calories: 118 |Carbs: 20g |Total Fat: 2g |Protein: 4g

Baked Oatmeal with Spiralized Apples

Upgrade your morning oatmeal with this spiralized apple recipe! It's top with honeycrisp apples noodles and crunchy walnuts.

Prep Time: 10 Minutes
Cook Time: 40 Minutes
Total Time: 50 Minutes
Yields: 1 -2 Servings

Ingredients:

- 1 honey-crisp apple, peeled and spiralized
- 2 large eggs
- 1 ¾ cups almond milk
- 1/3 cup maple syrup
- 3 Tbsp. melted coconut oil, divided
- 2 cups old-fashioned oats
- 2 tsp. vanilla extract
- 2 tsp. ground cinnamon
- 1 tsp. baking powder
- ¼ tsp. ground nutmeg
- ¾ tsp. fine-grain sea salt
- 2/3 cup roughly chopped walnuts

Directions:

1. Preheat the oven to 375 degrees F
2. Grease a 10" skillet or 9" baking dish
3. In a medium bowl, add the oats, walnuts, cinnamon, baking powder, salt and nutmeg, whisk well to combine
4. In a smaller bowl, add the milk, maple syrup, egg, half of the coconut oil, and vanilla, whisk until blended
5. Spiralize the apple with a small blade
6. Reserve half of the apple for topping the baked oatmeal, then arrange the rest of the apples evenly over the bottom of the baking dish
7. Cover the top of the apples with the dry oat mixture, then drizzle the wet ingredients on top of the oats, gently shake the baking dish to make sure the almond milk moves down through the oats, then pat down the dry oats resting on top
8. Sprinkle the rest of the apple noodles on top
9. Bake for 35 to 45 minutes, until the top of the oatmeal is brown and crisp, if any of the apple noodles start to burn, tuck them into the oatmeal or snip them off

10. Remove the baked oatmeal from the oven and allow it to cool for a few minutes
11. Drizzle the remaining coconut oil on the top before serving, if desired
12. Serve!

Nutritional Facts Per Serving |Calories: 425 |Carbs: 52g |Total Fat: 22g |Protein: 13g

Cheddar and Broccoli Egg Muffins

Instead of ordinary baked muffins, opt to make these fluffy egg muffins that are packed with cheddar and fresh broccoli!

Prep Time: 10 Minutes
Cook Time: 20 Minutes
Total Time: 30 Minutes
Yields: 12 Muffins

Ingredients:

- 1 cup chopped broccoli florets
- 2 large broccoli stems, spiralized, noodles trimmed
- 14 large eggs
- ¼ cup shredded cheddar cheese

Directions:

1. Preheat the oven to 400 degrees F
2. Grease the muffin tin with olive oil cooking spray
3. Spiralize the broccoli with a small blade, trim and set aside
4. In a medium bowl, beat the eggs
5. In each muffin tin, add about 1/3 of the way with a mix of broccoli noodles and florets
6. In each cavity, use a ladle and pour over the eggs to fill three-quarters of the way to the top, sprinkle with the shredded cheese, about a teaspoon for each muffin
7. Bake for 15 to 20 minutes or until the eggs are set completely
8. Remove from the oven
9. Allow the muffins to cool for a couple of minutes or until ready to handle
10. Serve immediately!

Nutritional Facts Per Serving |Calories: 105 |Carbs: 2g |Total Fat: 7g |Protein: 9g

Appetizers

Crisp Cornmeal Veggie Fritters

Kick off the party with these Crispy Cornmeal Veggie Fritters that are surprisingly tasty and healthy!

Prep Time: 10 Minutes
Cook Time: 10 Minutes
Total Time: 20 Minutes
Yields: 4-6 Servings

Ingredients:

- 1 large carrot, peeled and spiralized, trimmed
- 1 large zucchini, peeled and spiralized noodles, trimmed
- 5 scallions, chopped
- 2 eggs, beaten
- ¾ cup organic corn meal
- 1 tsp. tumeric
- 2 Tbsp. olive oil
- Salt, to taste
- Pepper, to taste

Directions:

1. Slice your carrot and zucchini half-way through, lengthwise, then spiralize (small blade)
2. In a large bowl, add the spiralized carrots, zucchini, scallions, cornmeal, salt, pepper, turmeric, and eggs, mix until thoroughly combined.
3. Place a skillet over medium heat, add ½ Tbsp. of olive oil
4. Once heated, scoop out about ¼ - ½ cup of the mixture
5. Place it on to one side of the pan and then flatten the mixture with a spatula so it resembles a small patty, repeat and place on the other side of the pan
6. Cook until crisp for about 2 to 3 minutes, flip over, then gently flatten with the spatula and cook for another 2 to 3 minutes or until a patty is formed and crispy
7. Repeat with the remaining mixture
8. Serve!

Nutritional Facts Per Serving |Calories: 152 |Carbs: 20g |Total Fat: 7g | Protein: 5g

Bacon Potato Home Fries

There's nothing like home fries! And this super fast 20 minute recipe will help you spend less time in the kitchen and more time with your guests.

Prep Time: 10 Minutes
Cook Time: 10 Minutes
Total Time: 20 Minutes
Yields: 3-4

Ingredients:

- 3 slices of bacon
- ½ Tbsp. extra virgin olive oil
- 1 large waxy potatoes, peeled, spiralized ribbons, trimmed
- 1 tsp. smoked paprika
- ½ tsp. garlic powder
- ¼ tsp. onion powder
- Coarse sea salt, to taste
- Pepper, to taste
- 1 Tbsp. of minced parsley, to garnish

Toppings:

- Sour cream
- Avocado slices
- Jalopeno

Directions:

1. Place a large skillet over medium heat, spray with cooking spray or oil
2. Once heated, add the bacon slices, cook until crispy, about 3 to 4 minute, set the cooked bacon on a paper towel-lined plate and keep all the bacon fat in the skillet, set on top of the stove
3. Place the potato ribbons into a large bowl, add in the olive oil and toss thoroughly to coat, then season with paprika, onion powder, garlic powder, salt and pepper.
4. Once again heat the skillet with the bacon fat grease over medium heat
5. Once heated add the potato noodles to the bacon fat, toss, and cover, cook for 7 to 10 minutes, or until the potato noodles are thoroughly cooked, uncover occasionally to toss the noodles, then cover again to continue cooking
6. When the noodles are done, crumble the bacon and add to skillet, toss and divide among the plates
7. Garnish with parsley and the toppings of choice
8. Serve!

Nutritional Facts Per Serving |Calories: 161 |Carbs: 23g |Total Fat: 6g |Protein: 6g

Prosciutto Wrapped Maple-Balsamic Sweet Potato Noodle Rolls

Serve your guests these crowd-pleasing Prosciutto Wrapped Maple-Balsamic Sweet Potato Noodle Rolls at a casual brunch or dinner with family and friends!

Prep Time: 15 Minutes
Cook Time: 5 Minutes
Total Time: 20 Minutes
Yields: 12 Rolls

Ingredients:

- 1 large sweet potato, peeled, spiralized noodles
- 12 slices of prosciutto, sliced in half
- 3 Tbsp. goat cheese
- 6 dates, pitted and sliced thinly
- ½ cup chopped pecans

For the maple-balsamic glaze:

- ¼ cup maple syrup
- 3 Tbsp. balsamic vinegar
- 2 tsp. Dijon mustard

Directions:

1. Place a large skillet over medium heat, add in the olive oil
2. Once heated, add in the sweet potato noodles and season with salt and pepper. Cover and cook the noodles for 5 to 7 minutes, uncovering to toss occasionally, until noodles soften and cook through
3. In the meantime, pour the syrup and vinegar into a small saucepan, whisk to combine and then bring to a boil. Cook until it reduces to 1/3 cup, about 3 to 5 minutes, stirring occasionally
4. Once the sauce has reduced, remove from heat and stir in the mustard, then set aside
5. Place two pieces of prosciutto out and smear with ½ Tbsp. of goat cheese, then sprinkle with about 1 Tbsp. of pecans and then sliced dates from about 1 date
6. Next lay out a layer of sweet potato noodles, roll the prosciutto to create a wrap
7. Slice in half and secure with a toothpick
8. Repeat with remaining prosciutto, to create 6 rolls in total, if you would like your appetizer larger then don't slice in half
9. Arrange the rolls on a serving platter and drizzle each the maple-balsamic
10. Serve!

Nutritional Facts Per Serving | Calories: 167 | Carbs: 17g |Total Fat: 8g | Protein: 10g

Zucchini Pesto Caprese Bites

Light and delicious, these little Zucchini Pesto Caprese Bites are the perfect appetizers before an Italian inspired dish.

Prep Time: 15 Minutes
Total Time: 15 Minutes
Yields: 6 Bites

Ingredients:

- ½ medium zucchini, spiralized ribbons, trimmed
- 2 Tbsp. pesto sauce
- 6 ¼" thick round slices of mozzarella, halved
- 1 beefsteak tomato, sliced into 3 ¼" thick round slices, halved
- Olive oil, to drizzle
- Salt, to taste
- Pepper, to taste

Directions:

1. In a medium bowl, toss the zucchini ribbon noodles with the pesto until thoroughly covered
2. Prepare the bites by placing one half mozzarella slice down on a clean surface, then add on a tomato slice
3. Carefully roll up some zucchini noodles and layer on top
4. Finish the bites with another mozzarella slice, repeat until all ingredients are used
5. Transfer to a serving platter
6. Optional drizzle with olive oil, salt, and pepper
7. Serve

Nutritional Facts Per Serving |Calories: 107 |Carbs: 2g |Total Fat: 8g |Protein: 6g

Sweet Potato Fries

Ready in just 30 minutes, you can season these spiralized sweet potato fries with everything from Cajun spice to jerk spices, and even cinnamon and sugar for your guests!

Prep Time: 10 Minutes
Cook Time: 20 Minutes
Total Time: 30 Minutes
Yields: 4 Servings

Ingredients:

- 1 medium sweet potato peeled, sprialized noodles
- 2 Tbsp. corn flour
- 1 Tbsp. rapeseed oil plus extra for greasing
- Salt, to taste
- Pepper, to taste

Seasoning Options:

- Jerk spices
- Cajun spices
- Cinnamon and sugar
- Dried herbs

Directions:

1. Preheat oven to 400 degrees F
2. Lightly grease the baking tray with oil
3. Thickly spiralize the sweet potatoes
4. In a large bowl, gently toss the sweet potato with the corn flour, add the oil and toss to coat
5. Spread the noodles over the baking tray or cooking mesh, making sure not to overcrowd. Use another baking tray if necessary
6. Bake for 20 minutes, turn the sweet potatoes halfway through and turn the trays, the fries will continue to crisp after they are removed from the oven
7. Seasoned with salt and pepper
8. Serve!

Nutritional Facts Per Serving |Calories: 74 |Carbs: 10g |Total Fat: 3g |Protein: 0g

Vietnamese Spring Rolls

Enjoy Vietnamese Spring Rolls, but with an even healthier twist! This recipe makes 12 spring rolls that are filled fresh vegetables and shrimp.

Prep Time: 20 Minutes
Total Time: 20 Minutes
Yields: 12 Rolls

Ingredients:

- 1 lb. cooked peeled shrimp, deveined and
- 12 spring roll skins
- 2 large zucchini, spiralized noodles, trimmed
- 1 cup shredded carrots
- 1 red bell pepper, thinly sliced
- 1 bunch basil leaves
- 1 bunch green onions, sliced
- ½ tsp. salt
- ¼ tsp. garlic powder
- ¼ tsp. cayenne pepper

Directions:

1. Fill a cake pan with water, set aside
2. Place the shrimp in a bowl, season with salt, garlic powder and cayenne pepper, toss to coat, make sure the tails are removed
3. Spiralize the zucchini into long noodles trim and, set aside
4. Cut the green onions into thin 1 ½ inch ribbons, set aside
5. Use a veggie peeler or knife to slice the red pepper into strips, set aside
6. One at a time, dip the spring roll skins into water, holding them in the water for about 10 seconds
7. then lay the spring roll skin out flat and top with 2 to 3 shrimp, followed by the basil leaves
8. Add a small portion of each veggies (green onion, zucchini, carrots and red peppers) over the top
9. Fold one end of the spring roll wrapper over the filling, pull tight and roll, tucking the end under as you roll
10. Place on a plate and repeat with the remaining ingredients
11. Once done, serve as-is or with soy sauce, or peanut sauce

Nutritional Facts Per Serving |Calories: 95 |Carbs: 13.3g |Total Fat: 0.7g |Protein: 9g

Chili Cheese Spiralized Fries

Make your guests happy while they wait for the main dish with a bowl of spiralized fries covered with homemade chili and yummy toppings!

Prep Time: 20 Minutes
Cook Time: 30 Minutes
Total Time: 50 Minutes
Yields: 6 Servings

Ingredients:

- 1 Tbsp. olive oil
- ½ lb. organic lean ground turkey or beef
- 1 small jalapeño, seeded and minced
- 1 (14.5 oz.) can red kidney beans or black beans, drained and rinsed
- 1 (14.5 oz.) can diced tomatoes, no salt added
- ½ small red onion, diced, about ½ cup
- ¼ cup carrots, diced, about 2 small carrots
- ¼ cup celery, dice, about 1 celery stalk
- 1 large garlic clove, minced
- 2 medium sweet potatoes
- ½ cup chicken broth, low sodium
- 2 tsp. dried oregano
- 1 - 1 ½ Tbsp. chili powder
- ½ tsp. ground cumin
- 1 bay leaf
- Salt, to taste
- Pepper, to taste

Toppings:

- 2 cups shredded cheddar cheese
- ½ cup diced scallions, to garnish
- Jalapeño
- Sour cream

Directions:

1. Preheat the oven to 425 degrees F and line two baking sheets with parchment paper
2. Prepare the chili by placing a large pot over medium heat, add the oil
3. Once heated, add in the turkey meat, season with salt and pepper, and cook while breaking it up into bits

4. When the meat is cooked and crumbled, add in the jalapeño, onion, carrots, celery, chili powder, garlic, oregano, cumin and stir well, cook for about 5 minutes or until softened
5. Add the chicken broth, tomatoes, bay leaf, and season with salt and pepper and then raise the heat to high and bring to a boil.
6. Once boiling, reduce the heat to medium-low and allow the chili to simmer, stirring occasionally, for about 20 minutes or until it thickened,
7. Add in the beans halfway through, once thickened and cooked, taste and adjust the seasoning with more salt if needed
8. Spiralize the sweet potatoes into noodles and then lay them out on the baking sheets, spray with olive oil cooking spray and season with salt and pepper.
9. Bake for 12 to 15 minutes or until wilted and al dente, then remove the pan from the oven and set aside.
10. Once the chili and sweet potatoes are done, pour the chili over the sweet potato noodles (on the baking sheets) and sprinkle with the cheese, then return the baking sheet to the oven and bake for an additional 5 minutes or until cheese melts
11. Once cooked, plate the chili fries and garnish with the toppings of your choice, enjoy!

Nutritional Facts Per Serving |Calories: 304 | Carbs: 25g |Total Fat: 14g |Protein: 21g

Potato Waffles with Chorizo and Parsley

Prep Time: 15 Minutes
Cook Time: 20 Minutes
Total Time: 35 Minutes
Yields: 2 Servings

Ingredients:

- 2.25 oz. chorizo, de-cased and crumbled
- 1 large red potato, peeled, spiralize noodles, roughly trimmed
- ¼ tsp. garlic powder
- Salt and pepper, to taste
- 1 large egg
- ¼ tsp. smoked paprika
- 1 tsp. minced parsley
- Maple syrup, to drizzle
- Mash avocado

Directions:

1. Preheat a Belgian waffle iron
2. In the meantime, place a large skillet over medium heat
3. Once heated, add in the chorizo and cook for 5 to7 minutes or until lightly browned
4. Once done, set the chorizo on a plate, then add in the potato noodles and season with garlic powder, salt and pepper, then cover and cook for 5 minutes or until the noodles have wilted and cooked through, tossing occasionally
5. Then transfer the noodles to a large mixing bowl with the chorizo and allow it to cool for two minutes Add in the egg, smoked paprika and parsley, toss to combine fully
6. Spray the waffle iron with cooking spray and then add in the potato mixture
7. Cook according to the waffle iron's settings for about 7 minutes, then remove carefully
8. Serve the waffles topped with maple syrup

Nutritional Facts Per Serving |Calories: 244 |Carbs: 15 g |Total Fat:15 g |Protein:13 g

Meatballs in Potato Noodle Cups with Tomato Sauce

Want to spend less time in the kitchen during your dinner party? Then quickly whip up these delicious Meatballs in Potato Noodle Cups with Tomato Sauce that will be ready in no time.

Prep Time: 15 Minutes
Cook Time: 30 Minutes
Total Time: 45 Minutes
Yields: 6 Servings

Ingredients:

- 1 Tbsp. extra virgin olive oil
- 6 pre-cooked meatballs, defrosted
- ¾ cup jarred tomato sauce
- 2 large russet potatoes, peeled, spiralized noodles, trimmed
- ½ tsp. garlic powder
- 2 large eggs, beaten
- Salt, to taste
- Pepper, to taste

Directions:

1. Preheat the oven to 425 degrees F
2. Grease a large muffin tin with cooking spray
3. In a large skillet over medium-high heat, add the oil
4. Once heated, add in the potato noodles, season with salt, pepper and garlic powder, toss and cook for 7 to 10 minutes or until cooked through and lightly browned
5. Transfer the potato noodles to a medium mixing bowl, allow to cool for 2 minutes
6. Add the eggs to the bowl and toss thoroughly to combine
7. Pack the potato noodles into the muffin holes, creating a cavity in the center
8. Bake for 15 minutes or until potato mixture has set
9. While the potato cups bake, pour the tomato sauce into a small skillet over medium heat and bring to a simmer, add in the meatballs and allow them to cook through while the potato cups cook
10. Once the potato cups are finished, remove and place on a platter
11. Place a meatball on top of each potato cup, top with extra sauce, if desired
12. Serve!

Nutritional Facts Per Serving |Calories: 136 |Carbs: 8g |Total Fat: 9g |Protein: 7g

Garlic Asiago Baked Spiralized Potatoes Fries

Instantly spice up your party when you pass out these Garlic Asiago Baked Spiralized Potatoes!

Prep Time: 10 Minutes
Cook Time: 25 Minutes
Total Time: 35 Minutes
Yields: 4 Servings

Ingredients:

- 1 medium sweet potato, spiralized, trimmed
- 1 medium Idaho potato, spiralized, trimmed
- 2 Tbsp. extra virgin olive oil
- 1 Tbsp. garlic powder
- 1/3 cup grated asiago cheese
- Fine sea salt, to taste
- Ground pepper, to taste

Directions:

1. Preheat the oven to 450 degrees F
2. Line a baking tray with nonstick parchment paper, set aside
3. Cut the potato noodles so that they length is serving friendly
4. In a mixing bowl, add in the potato noodles, drizzle with the olive oil, toss, then add in the garlic powder, asiago cheese and season with salt and pepper, generously. Toss to coat
5. Lay the potatoes out on the prepared baking tray, making sure not to overlap the potatoes. Prepare another baking tray
6. Sprinkle with the rest of the asiago cheese, careful to cover all potatoes
7. Bake in the oven for 10 to 15 minutes and then flip over, bake for another 10 to 15 minutes or until browned, flipping every 5 minutes if necessary
8. Remove from the oven
9. Divide into small bowls and serve!

Nutritional Facts Per Serving |Calories: 159 |Carbs: 15g |Total Fat: 10g |Protein: 4g

Veggie and Sun-Dried Tomato Pesto Pizza

Change things up and serve a pizza as the appetizer instead of the main dish! This pizza is topped with spiralized veggie like carrots, yellow squash and zucchini.

Prep Time: 5 Minutes
Cook Time: 10 Minutes
Total Time: 15 Minutes
Yields: 6-8 Servings

Ingredients:

- 1 large, thick carrot, peeled, spiralized
- 1 medium zucchini, spiralized
- 1 medium yellow squash, spiralized
- 1 pre-made thin crust Italian pizza crust
- ½ cup Sun-Dried Tomato Pesto sauce
- 8 oz. fresh mozzarella, sliced ¼-inch thick
- ½ small red onion, thinly sliced
- ½ cup shredded Parmesan cheese

Directions:

1. Preheat the oven to 450 degrees F
2. Using the spiralizer, make thin spirals of zucchini, carrot and yellow squash, yield about 1 cup of each Place all the vegetable spirals between two layers of paper towels and gently squeeze to remove as much moisture as possible, set aside.
3. Spread the Sun-Dried Tomato Pesto in an even layer over the pre-made pizza crust
4. Place the mozzarella slices over pesto, arrange spiralized vegetables evenly over cheese
5. Sprinkle on the red onion slices
6. Top with the Parmesan cheese
7. Place pizza directly on oven rack
8. Bake until cheese is melted and crust is browned, about 8 to 10 minutes
9. Serve

Nutritional Facts Per Serving (minus the pre-made crust of your choice) |Calories: 169 |Carbs: 11.76g |Total Fat: 3.83g |Protein: 23.41g

Bacon Zucchini Fritters

Quickly make these savory bacon zucchini fritters that are packed with veggies and so addicting! Just serve them with homemade ranch or mayo.

Prep Time: 35 minutes
Cook Time: 10 minutes
Total Time: 45 minutes
Servings: 16 fritters

Ingredients:

- 4 cups zucchini, spiralized noodle, trimmed short
- ¾ tsp. salt, to "sweat" the zucchini
- 6 Slices Bacon
- 2 Tbsp. coconut flour
- 2-3 Tbsp. cooking fat, rendered bacon fat, ghee, or coconut oil
- 2 Tbsp. arrowroot flour
- 1 large egg, whisked
- ½ tsp. onion powder
- ¼ tsp. garlic powder
- ¼ - ½ tsp. black pepper

For Dipping:

- Ranch
- Chipotle Ranch
- Mayo

Directions:

1. Sweat the zucchini by placing it in a colander, then place the colander over a bowl, sprinkle with the salt and allow it to sit for about 20 minutes - the longer it sits, the more water is drawn out. After 20 minute or longer, gently rinse zucchini to remove excess salt.
2. Using a paper towel or clean dish towel, squeeze or wring out the remaining water to avoid having very soggy fritters, set aside
3. Place a large skillet over medium heat, add the bacon and cook for 5-7 minutes or until crispy, then drain and crumble, set aside - if desired reserve 2 Tbsp. of the fat for frying the fritters
4. In a large bowl, mix together the prepared zucchini, crumbled bacon, coconut flour, arrowroot, egg, onion powder, garlic powder, pepper and salt to taste
5. Place a large skillet over medium heat, then add 1 Tbsp. cooking fat
6. Scoop the fritter mixture in heaping tablespoon (or cookie scoop) into a hot skillet and gently press down to about 1/2" thickness

7. Cook for about 2 to 3 minutes, until the first side is golden brown, then flip and fry on the second side for 2 to 3 minutes until golden brown, lower the heat if necessary
8. Repeat with the remaining mixture and add an additional Tbsp. cooking fat before each new batch
9. Serve hot with your favorite dipping sauce

Nutritional Facts Per Serving |Calories: 66 |Carbs: 2g |Total Fat: 5g |Protein: 1g

Spicy Roasted Spiralized Sweet Potatoes with Guacamole

Your guests (and you) will absolutely love having Spicy Roasted Sweet Potato Spirals top with zesty homemade guacamole as an appetizer.

Prep Time: 20 Minutes
Cook Time: 50 Minutes
Total Time: 1 Hour 10 Minutes
Yields: 4 Servings

Ingredients:

- 3 medium sweet potatoes, spiralized noodles
- Hot water plus 1 tsp. salt
- 2 Tbsp. olive oil
- 1 tsp. garlic powder
- ½ tsp. chilli powder
- ½ tsp. cumin
- 1 tsp. salt
- Guacamole

Garnish:

- Green onion, diced
- Lime wedges

Directions:

1. Preheat the oven to 475 degrees F
2. In a large bowl, soak the sweet potato spirals in hot salt water for 15 minutes, remove from the water and pat the spirals dry, making sure you remove as much of the moisture as possible
3. Place the spirals in a dry bowl, toss with the olive oil and seasonings until well coated
4. Arrange the spiralized sweet potatoes on lined sheet
5. Bake for 50 to 60 minutes, toss every 20 minutes, until they reach crunchiness you desire
6. Served topped with guacamole and garnish with green onions and lime wedges

Nutritional Facts Per Serving |Calories: 149 |Carbs: 20.75g |Total Fat: 6.98g |Protein: 1.73g

Vegetarians and Vegans

Butternut Noodles with Garlic Mushrooms and Lentils

Served with a creamy white sauce, this comforting pasta dish is made with spiralized butternut squash, mushrooms, lentils and aromatic sage.

Prep Time: 2 Minutes
Cook Time: 8 Minutes
Total Time: 10 Minutes
Yields: 2 Servings

Ingredients:

- 1 Tbsp. olive oil
- 1 medium butternut squash, peeled and spiralized noodles
- 10 white cup mushrooms, peeled and sliced
- ½ cup precooked lentils
- Few fresh sage leaves, roughly chopped

The Creamy Sauce

- ½ cup unsweetened almond milk
- 1 Tbsp. arrowroot powder or tapioca flour
- ½ tsp. garlic powder or 2 garlic cloves, minced
- 4 Tbsp. nutritional yeast flakes

Directions:

1. In a large saucepan or wok over medium heat, add the olive oil
2. Once heated, add the butternut noodles until they begin to soften, about 2 to 3 minutes
3. Add in the mushrooms, lentils and sage, cook for another 5 minutes
4. Prepare the sauce by mixing the almond milk and arrowroot together in a small bowl, then add to pan along with the garlic powder or minced garlic, stir into the noodles. As the sauce cooks it will begin to thicken
5. Once the sauce becomes thick and creamy, remove from the heat and stir in the nutritional flakes.
6. Season with salt and pepper to taste
7. Enjoy!

Nutritional Facts Per Serving |Calories: 241 |Carbs: 24g |Total Fat: 9g |Protein: 13.5g

Recipe Notes:

- This is a vegan pasta dish, you can opt to make it non vegan by replacing the almond milk with regular milk and the nutritional yeast with cheese.

Sweet Potato Enchilada Skillet

Everything you love about enchiladas, but much healthier! This 30-minute skillet version is made with spiralized sweet potato noodles, sweet corn, black beans, and gooey cheese.

Prep Time: 10 Minutes
Cook Time: 20 Minutes
Total Time: 30 Minutes
Yields: 6 Servings

Ingredients:

1 Tbsp. olive oil
1 small onion
11 oz. of sweet potato, peeled, spiralized noodles
2 cloves garlic, minced
1 can black beans (9 oz.) drained and rinsed
1 can corn kernels (12 oz.) drained and rinsed
4 6-inch corn tortillas cut into ½ inch strips, or flour tortillas
2 cups enchilada sauce
2 cups of Mexican cheese blend, divided

To serve:

- Cilantro
- Avocado
- Greek yogurt

Directions:

1. Pre-heat oven to 350 degrees F
2. In a large oven proof skillet (12 inches) over medium heat, add the olive oil
3. Once heated, add in the onion and cook for 5 or until translucent and soft
4. Add in the sweet potato noodles, and cook for 10 or until al dente - they noodles should have a bite to them and not be too soft
5. Add in the garlic and cook for one minute
6. Then add in the black beans, corn, tortillas, enchilada sauce and half of the cheese, stir to completely combined
7. Sprinkle with the remaining cheese and place in the oven for 5 or so minutes, until the cheese is melted and the enchilada sauce bubbles
8. Serve with optional toppings listed.

Nutritional Facts Per Serving Size: 1/6 cup |Calories: 430 |Carbs: 58g |Total Fat:18g |Protein:20g

Recipe Note:

- Make this dish vegan by replacing the mozzarella cheese with plant-based mozzarella cheese and a yogurt that is also vegan (made with coconut, soy, almond, hemp, flax, or cashew milk.)

Coconut Curry Soup with Sweet Potato Noodles

Full of flavor, this easy-to-make Coconut Curry Soup with sweet potato noodles is perfect for lunch or as a light vegetarian dinner.

Prep Time: 10 Minutes
Cook Time: 22 Minutes
Total Time: 32 Minutes
Yields: 4 Servings

Ingredients:

- 1 large sweet potato, spiralized
- 1 small white onion, diced
- 3 cloves garlic, minced
- 1 Tbsp. minced fresh ginger
- 1 red bell pepper, cut into thin strips
- 2 Tbsp. yellow curry powder
- 3 cups low-sodium vegetable broth
- 1 (13.5 oz.) can coconut milk, full fat or light
- ½ cup frozen green peas
- Juice of 1/2 lime

Garnishes:

- Lime wedges
- Cilantro, if desired

Directions:

1. Preheat the oven to 425 degrees F
2. Arrange the spiralized sweet potato noodles on a rimmed baking sheet in a single layer
3. Bake for 10 minutes
4. In the meantime, place a soup pot over medium heat
5. Add the diced onions and sauté with 3 tbsp of water, until tender for about 5 to 6 minutes
6. Add the garlic, ginger, and red bell pepper and sauté for 2 minutes
7. Add the curry powder, vegetable broth, and coconut milk, simmer over medium heat for 15 to 20 minutes
8. Lastly, add in the green peas and lime juice, stir to combine

9. Ladle the soup into individual portions in bowls and then top with sweet potato noodles, lime juice and a sprinkle of the optional chopped cilantro

Nutritional Facts Per Serving |Calories: 268 |Carbs: 29g |Total Fat: 18g |Protein: 4g

Roasted Carrot Noodle Salad with Thyme Vinaigrette

Enjoy a colorful and delicious Roasted Carrot Noodle salad for lunch! This salad features tender, caramelized roasted carrot noodles tossed with a savory-sweet thyme vinaigrette.

Prep Time: 10 Minutes
Cook Time: 25 Minutes
Total Time: 35 Minutes
Yields: 4 Servings

Ingredients:

- 1 ½ - 2 lbs. carrots trimmed, peeled and spiralized, about 8 large carrots
- 1 bunch radishes assorted colors or pink, thinly sliced
- 1 bunch watercress stemmed
- ½ cup slivered almonds, toasted

Dressing:

- 1/3 cup extra virgin olive oil plus more for carrots
- 2 Tbsp. champagne vinegar or white wine vinegar
- 2 Tbsp. honey plus more for carrots
- 1 Tbsp. thyme leaves plus more for carrots, roughly chopped
- Salt, to taste
- Pepper, to taste

Optional Toppings:

- Plain yogurt
- Lemon wedges
- Crushed red pepper flakes
- Micro greens

Directions:

1. Preheat oven to 375 degrees F
2. Line a large, rimmed baking sheet with non-stick aluminum foil
3. Place the spiralized carrot noodles on the baking sheet and gently toss the with 1 ½ Tbsp. of oil, 2 tsp. of thyme and 1 tsp. of honey.
4. Then season with ¾ tsp. salt and ¼ tsp. pepper and cover the baking sheet tightly with another sheet of aluminum foil.

5. Roast in the oven for 10 minutes, or until steamed slightly, then uncover, discard of the foil and roast for an additional 10 to 15 minutes, or until the carrots are tender
6. In the meantime, prepare the vinaigrette by taking an empty jar with a tight-fitting lid and combine 1/3 cup of oil with vinegar, 2 Tbsp. honey, 1 Tbsp. thyme, and a dash of each salt and pepper. Close and shake the jar vigorously to emulsify, then adjust the seasoning with salt and pepper and sweetness with honey
7. Transfer roasted carrot noodles to a large serving bowl, add the radishes, gently toss with radishes and drizzle with 2 Tbsp. of the vinaigrette into the bowl, toss again to combine
8. Add in the watercress and toss to coat
9. Divide the carrot noodles evenly among plates and top with additional radishes, almonds and desired garnishes
10. Serve with the remaining vinaigrette on the side and enjoy!

Nutritional Facts Per Serving Size: cup |Calories: 321 |Carbs: 23g |Total Fat: 24g |Protein: 4g

Recipe Note:

- Make this recipe vegan friendly by replacing the honey with agave nectar, coconut nectar or maple syrup and choosing a plant or nut-based yogurt

Yellow Squash Pasta with Caramelized Lemon

In the mood for pasta dinner? Then whip up this bright Yellow Squash Pasta dish that's tossed with savory caramelized lemons, Parmigiano-Reggiano cheese and olive oil.

Prep Time: 20 Minutes
Cook Time: 3 Hours
Total Time: 3 Hours 20 Minutes
Yields: 4 Servings

Ingredients:

- 1 ½ lbs. yellow squash, about 3 large squash, spiralzied
- 3 medium lemons, divided
- 1 ½ Tbsp. olive oil, divided
- ½ cup roughly chopped celery leaves
- ¾ oz. Parmigiano-Reggiano cheese, finely grated (about ¼ cup)
- ½ tsp. black pepper
- ¼ tsp. kosher salt, divided
- 1/8 tsp. sugar

Directions:

1. Trim the squash on the ends, and cut the squash crosswise into halves, using a spoon, carefully scoop out inner seeds from each squash and remove as little flesh as possible. Use a spiralizer to create large noodles.
2. Place the squash noodles between 2 layers of paper towels, allow them to stand at room temperature until dry, about 3 hours
3. Transfer the noodles to a medium bowl, and grate the rind from 1 lemon to equal ½ tsp.
4. Cut same lemon in half, squeeze out the juice to have 1 Tbsp., then set aside the rind and juice. Prepare the other 2 lemons by trimming the tops and bottoms and slice into half-moons
5. Place a large nonstick skillet over medium-high, add 1 ½ tsp. of oil
6. Add lemon slices, sprinkle evenly with 1/8 tsp. of salt and sprinkle the sugar over lemons
7. Cook, stirring occasionally, until lemons start to brown around the edges and caramelized, 4 to 5 minutes
8. Add the caramelized lemon slices to squash noodles
9. Add in the celery leaves, cheese, lemon rind, lemon juice, pepper, and the remaining 1/8 tsp. of salt, toss gently to combine
10. Drizzle with remaining oil
11. Serve!

Nutritional Facts Per Serving |Calories: 97 |Carbs: 6g |Total Fat: 7.9g |Protein: 2g

Mediterranean Beet and Feta Skillet Bake

Fresh beet noodles baked with tomatoes, red onion, olives and topped with feta. Serve this skillet bake as a vegetarian main dish with a side of baked pita chips!

Prep Time: 10 Minutes
Cook Time: 20 Minutes
Total Time: 30 Minutes
Yields: 4 Servings

Ingredients:

- ½ cup halved yellow cherry tomatoes
- ½ cup halved yellow red tomatoes
- 2 medium cloves garlic, minced
- 2 Tbsp. minced fresh parsley, plus 1 tsp. for garnish
- 1 tsp. dried oregano
- 1 Tbsp. red wine vinegar
- 1 Tbsp. extra virgin olive oil
- 10 pitted Kalamata olives
- 2 small beets, peeled and spiralized noodles
- ½ small onion, peeled and spiralized noodles
- Kosher salt and black pepper, to taste
- 4 oz. feta or halloumi cheese, half block cut horizontally

Directions:

1. Preheat the oven to 400 degrees F
2. Using your spiralizer, spiralize the beets and small onions, set aside
3. In a large bowl, combine the cherry tomatoes, red tomatoes, minced garlic, minced parsley, oregano, red wine vinegar, extra virgin olive oil, spiralized beets and spiralized onion, season with salt and black pepper
4. Place the cheese in the center of a large oven-safe skillet or casserole dish, top and surround it with beet noodle mixture, and then cover the dish with foil
5. Bake for 20 minutes, until the beet noodles wilt
6. Serve garnished with remaining parsley

Nutritional Facts Per Serving (¼ of recipe) |Calories: 160.5 |Carbs: 9g |Total Fat: 12g |Protein: 5g

Stir-Fry Zucchini Noodles

This healthy vegetarian stir-fry is made with spiralized zucchini and onions tossed in your favorite teriyaki sauce and topped with toasted sesame seeds!

Prep Time: 10 Minutes
Cook Time: 10 Minutes
Total Time: 20 Minutes
Yields: 4 Servings

Ingredients:

- 2 Tbsp. vegetable oil
- 2 yellow onions, spiralized noodles
- 4 small zucchini, spiralized noodles, patted dry with paper towel
- 1 Tbsp. low-sodium soy sauce
- 2 Tbsp. low-sodium teriyaki sauce
- 1 Tbsp. sesame seeds

Directions:

1. Place a skillet or wok over medium heat, add the oil
2. Once heated add in the onions, cook for 4 to 5 minutes, or until translucent and tender
3. Stir in the zucchini and cook for 2 minutes
4. Add in the soy sauce, teriyaki sauce and sesame seeds, mix and continue to cook for 5 minutes, or until zucchini is tender
5. Once cooked, remove from heat
6. Serve!

Nutritional Facts Per Serving |Calories: 137 |Carbs: 13g |Total Fat: 8g |Protein: 4g

Creamy Roasted Tomato Basil Zucchini Noodle Soup

Enjoy fresh summer produce with this effortless soup recipe that features a creamy roasted tomato basil base with zucchini noodles!

Prep Time: 7 Minutes
Cook Time: 25 Minutes
Total Time: 32 Minutes
Yields: 2 Servings

Ingredients:

For the soup:

- 1 zucchini, spiralized noodles
- 10 campari tomatoes
- 1 cup vegetable broth, low-sodium
- 2 Tbsp. 0% non-fat plain Greek Yogurt
- 1 Tbsp. olive oil, plus more olive oil for drizzling
- 2 garlic cloves, minced
- 6 tsp. basil, finely chopped
- ½ cup chopped red onions
- Pepper grinder, to taste
- ¼ tsp. red pepper flakes, more if desired
- 2 slices of whole grain bread, optional (for dipping)

For the kale chips:

- 3-4 pieces of kale, washed and completely dry
- Olive oil, for drizzling
- 1/8 tsp. of garlic powder
- Sea salt grinder

Directions:

1. Preheat the oven to 375 degrees F
2. Slice the tomatoes in half and lay, flat sides up, on a baking tray, drizzle with olive oil and season with salt and pepper, then roast for 20 minutes
3. During the last 10 minutes, prepare the kale chips, coat a baking tray with cooking spray and arrange the dry kale, drizzle lightly with olive oil and rub the oil into the kale leaves by hand. Season the kale very lightly with salt and garlic powder
4. Place the kale into the oven for 5-7 minutes, watch them carefully after 4 minutes to make sure they don't burn. Once cooked, set aside
5. Place a large saucepan over medium-low heat, add in the olive oil
6. Once oil heats, add in the garlic and red pepper flakes and cook for 1 minute
7. Then add in the onions and cook for about 1 to 2 minutes or until soft

8. Once done, pour into a food processor, along with the tomatoes and any juices on the baking tray
9. Pour the puree back into the large saucepan, over medium heat, and add in the vegetable broth and chopped basil, bring the soup to a boil and then allow it simmer for 10 minutes
10. Add in the zucchini noodles and cook for 2 minutes
11. Once the noodles cooked, stir in the Greek Yogurt and simmer for another 1 minute
12. Pour the soup into bowls, top with kale chips, and serve with warmed bread of your choice

Nutritional Facts Per Serving |Calories: 409 |Carbs: 62 g |Total Fat: 16g |Protein: 13g
Nutritional Facts Per Serving | Calories: 29 |Carbs: 2.46 g |Total Fat: 0.52g |Protein: 2.46g

Loaded Veggie Pasta Salad with Sweet Basil Vinaigrette

Changes things up and combine wheat pasta with fresh zoodles to creat a filling loaded veggie pasta with a sweet basil vinaigrette. Yes, you will have to boil water, but it's worth it.

Prep Time: 10 Minutes
Cook Time: 8 Minutes
Total Time: 18 Minutes
Yields: 6 Servings

Ingredients:

- 1 Tbsp. olive oil
- 8 oz. whole wheat spaghetti
- 2 medium zucchini, spiralized
- 3 cloves garlic, minced
- 2 cups fresh or frozen peas, thawed
- 1 bunch thin asparagus, trimmed and cut into 1 ½-inch pieces
- ¼ cup freshly grated Parmesan cheese
- 4 slices bacon, cooked and crumbled

For the Sweet Basil Vinaigrette:

- ½ cup fresh basil leaves
- 2 Tbsp. white wine vinegar
- 2 tsp. Dijon mustard
- 2 tsp. honey
- 1 tsp. minced shallots
- ½ tsp. salt
- ¼ cup olive oil

Directions:

1. Place a large pot over medium heat, fill it with water and a dose of salt, and bring to boil
2. Cook the spaghetti according to package directions, drain and set aside
3. Prepare the vinaigrette by placing the basil, vinegar, Dijon mustard, honey, shallots, salt and olive oil in a blender, blend for about 30 seconds to a minute, set aside
4. In a large skillet over medium heat, drizzle in the olive oil and sauté garlic, peas and asparagus for about 3 to 5 minutes, until the garlic is fragrant and the veggies are tender
5. Then add in the zucchini noodles and cook an additional 1 to 2 minutes
6. In a large bowl toss together the zucchini noodles, warm spaghetti, veggies and Parmesan cheese with the basil vinaigrette
7. Top with crumbled bacon and enjoy!

Nutritional Facts Per Serving (¼ of the batch)| Calories: 229|Carbs: 23.2g |Total Fat: 12.1g |Protein: 9.2g

Apple Cranberry Salad

This 10 minutes spiralized Apple Cranberry Salad is made with crunchy, crisp apples, cranberries, pecans and goat cheese tossed in a refreshing citrus poppy seed dressing, for a healthy and delicious vegetarian entree!

Prep Time: 10 Minutes

Total Time: 10 Minutes

Yields 2-4

Ingredients:

- 1 red apple or pink lady
- 1 granny smith apple
- ¼ cup dried cranberries
- ¼ cup golden raisins
- ¼ cup crumbled goat cheese
- 1/3 cup pecans, chopped and toasted, optional
- ½ cup citrus poppy seed dressing

Citrus Poppy Seed Dressing:

- 1/3 cup olive oil
- ¼ cup lime, juiced
- ¼ cup champagne or apple cider vinegar
- 1 Tbsp. dijon mustard
- 2 Tbsp. dried onion
- 1 Tbsp. poppy seeds
- 6 Tbsp. honey
- 2 Tbsp. water
- ½ tsp. salt

Directions:

1. Prepare the dressing by combining the olive oil, lime juice, vinegar, Dijon mustard, dried onion, poppy seeds, honey, water and salt in a bowl, mix well to combine, then store in the fridge until ready to use
2. Spiralize the apples and toss with the dressing
3. Add in the dried cranberries, golden raisins, crumbled goat cheese and pecans
4. Serve!

Recipe Note:

- You can refrigerate the salad for up to 1 hour. If you opt to use store-bought poppy seed dressing, make a mixture of 2 parts poppy seed dressing to 1-part lemon or lime juice.

- Make this dish vegan by removing the goat cheese and replacing the honey with agave syrup or brown rice syrup.

Nutritional Facts Per Serving Size ½ cup |Calories: 523 |Carbs: 57g |Total Fat: 30g |Protein: 8g

Pesto Zoodle Salad

Enjoy a refreshing and unique summer salad that's made with zucchini and carrot noodles topped with sun dried tomatoes and an easy 3 ingredient pesto vinaigrette!

Prep Time: 15 Minutes
Cook Time: 12 Minutes
Total Time: 27 Minutes
Yields: 6 Servings

Ingredients:

- 2 zucchinis large, spiralized noodles
- 1 carrot large, peeled, spiralized noodles
- 1 cup black olives
- ¼ cup sun dried tomatoes
- 1 cup red cabbage, shredded
- 2 bell peppers, red & yellow
- 1 cup marinated artichoke hearts
- Olive oil

Pesto Vinaigrette:

- ¼ cup white wine vinegar
- ¼ cup lemon juice
- ¼ cup pesto

Toppings:

- Parmesan

Directions:

1. Prepare pesto vinaigrette by adding the white vinegar, lemon juice and pesto to a jar and then shake, set aside.
2. Preheat oven to broil on high, if you are making roasted peppers
3. Slice the peppers, and then place on a baking tray, lightly spray with olive oil and roast for 10 to 14 minutes, until the peppers start to char
4. Spiralize the zucchini and carrots, add to a large salad bowl, and then in add purple cabbage
5. Top with the rest of the salad with the black olives, sun dried tomatoes, marinated artichoke heart, roasted peppers and a drizzle of olive oil
6. Serve with the pesto vinaigrette and a sprinkle of Parmesan

Nutritional Facts Per Serving |Calories: 157 |Carbs: 13g |Total Fat: 10g |Protein: 3g

Avocado Spring Rolls

Want something fast and delicious for lunch? Then whip up these Avocado Spring Rolls that you can dip in a yummy peanut sauce.

Prep Time: 30 Minutes
Total Time: 30 Minutes
Yields: 6 Serving

Ingredients:

Spring rolls:

6 rice paper wrappers

- 1 large avocado, peeled, pitted and thinly sliced (1/8" thick)
- 1 large English seedless cucumber, spiralized, noodles trimmed
- 2 medium carrots, peeled and julienned
- 2 packed cups Boston or bibb lettuce
- Fresh cilantro, handful
- Fresh mint, handful
- 1 large lime, quartered
- Pepper, to taste

Dipping sauce:

- 1 tsp. sesame oil
- ¼ cup peanut oil
- ¼ cup tahini
- 3 Tbsp. soy sauce
- 2 Tbsp. red wine vinegar
- 2 tsp. chili oil
- 1 tsp. honey
- ½ tsp. cayenne pepper
- 1 garlic clove, minced

Directions:

1. Make the dipping sauce – combine the sesame oil, peanut oil, tahini, soy sauce, red wine vinegar, chili oil, honey cayenne pepper, and minced garlic all of the ingredients into a food processor and pulse until creamy. Reserve 6 tablespoons and save the rest in the refrigerator for later
2. Create a quick assembly line of the vegetables for the spring rolls
3. In a shallow dish, fill it with warm water
4. One at a time, dip a single rice wrapper sheet into the water for 5 to 10 seconds, remove and place on a cutting board or plate

5. In the middle of the rice wrapper, lay down 2 avocado slices down, 1 pinch of cilantro and 1 pinch of mint, the cucumber noodles, sliced carrots, and top with lettuce, squeeze over with 1/2 lime wedge and season with pepper
6. Wrap the rice paper wrapper by folding the bottom half of the rice paper wrapper over the filling, holding firmly in place, fold the sides of the wrapper in, and then press down firmly to hold it in place, roll the entire wrapper horizontally up from the bottom to the top
7. Turn the roll, making sure the seam faces down and the avocado faces up
8. Continue on with the remaining ingredients and rice wrappers to make four
9. Place on a plate and serve the spring rolls with the dipping sauce

Recipe Note:

- Make this vegan by replacing the honey with agave syrup, nectars or brown rice syrup. Cover with plastic wrap and refrigerate if you're not eating the spring rolls immediately

Nutritional Facts Per Serving |Calories: 176 |Carbs: 20g |Total Fat: 11g |Protein: 5g

Moroccan Spiralizer Carrot Rice

You won't miss plain white rice when you make this fragrant Moroccan Spiralized Carrot Rice!

Prep Time: 5 Minutes
Cook Time: 10 Minutes
Total Time: 15 Minutes
Yields: 4 Servings

Ingredients:

- 10 large carrots, peeled and spiralized grain-like
- 1 Tbsp. olive oil
- 1 tsp. garlic puree
- 1 tsp. ginger puree
- 1 tsp. cinnamon
- 1 tsp. turmeric
- 2 Tbsp. coriander
- Salt, to taste
- Pepper, to taste

Directions:

1. Using the Spiralizer, create thin carrot noodles
2. Place a wok or skillet over medium heat, add your garlic puree, carrots, olive oil and cook for 5 minutes
3. Add the cinnamon, turmeric, coriander, salt and pepper and cook for another 5 minutes
4. Place into a biscuit cutter to shape
5. Serve!

Nutritional Facts Per Serving |Calories: 102 |Carbs: 16g |Total Fat: 3g |Protein: 1g

Chipotle Sweet Potato Noodle Salad with Roasted Corn

Oh, you'll love making this easy Chipotle Sweet Potato Noodle Salad that's topped with a delicious chipotle garlic dressing and roasted corn!

Prep Time: 10 Minutes
Cook Time: 5 Minutes
Total Time: 15 Minutes
Yields: 4 Serving

Ingredients:

For the sweet potato noodle salad:

- Olive oil
- 2 sweet potatoes, spiralized
- 4 ears sweet corn (kernels cut off the cob)
- 1 cup chopped fresh cilantro
- 1 cup chopped fresh greens – spinach, micro greens, arugula, whatever
- ½ cup pepitas

For the chipotle dressing:

- 1/3 cup olive oil
- 2 individual chipotle peppers, canned in adobo sauce
- 3 Tbsp. water
- 1 clove garlic
- 1 tsp. agave or honey
- Juice of one orange
- Juice of one lemon or lime
- Generous pinch of salt

Directions:

1. Make the chipotle dressing by adding the olive oil, chipotle peppers, water, garlic clove, agave or honey, orange juice, lemon or lime juice and a pinch of salt to your food processor until combined and smooth, taste and adjust to your liking, set aside
2. In a skillet over medium heat, add a drizzle of olive oil
3. Add in the sweet potato noodles and toss for a minute or two until softened - making sure they don't overcook.
4. Remove the noodles and set aside
5. Wipe the skillet clean so it's dry
6. Place the skillet over medium high heat, add the corn kernels, toss occasionally for a few minutes until roasted
7. In a bowl, add the noodles, corn, cilantro, and pepitas, toss together - Set aside a little of each ingredient as a topping for the salad
8. Top with the chipotle dressing, toss to combine
9. Serve!

Nutritional Facts Per Serving |Calories: 322 |Carbs: 33g |Total Fat: 20.1g |Protein: 5.2g

Meat and Poultry

Honey Lemon Chicken Quinoa Bowls with Spiralized Veggies

So delicious and ready in just 30 minutes, this dish features stir-fry ground chicken in a sticky, tangy, sweet, honey lemon sauce on top of nutty quinoa and spiralized veggies!

Prep Time: 15 Minutes
Cook Time: 15 Minutes
Total Time: 30 Minutes
Yields: 4 Servings

Ingredients:

Stir-Fry:

- 1 lb. ground chicken
- Zucchini, spiralized noodles
- Squash, spiralized noodles
- 1 Tbsp. oil neutral flavored, vegetable or canola
- 1 small shallot, finely diced
- 2 tsp. ginger, freshly grated
- 2 cloves garlic, minced
- Kosher salt, to taste
- Ground black pepper, to taste

Sauce:

- 1 Tbsp. apple cider vinegar
- 1 Tbsp. cornstarch
- ½ cup unsalted chicken stock
- ¼ cup lemon juice, freshly squeezed
- 1 Tbsp. reduced sodium soy sauce
- Zest of 1 lemon
- 1/3 cup honey
- A pinch of crushed red pepper flakes or more to taste

Optional for serving

- Shredded lettuce
- Quinoa, (cooked according to package directions)
- Microgreens
- Sliced radishes
- Sliced green onions

- Sesame seeds
- Lemon wedges

Directions:

1. Prepare the sauce: In a small bowl, whisk together the apple cider vinegar, cornstarch, chicken stock, lemon juice, soy sauce, lemon zest, honey, and a pinch of sriracha or red pepper flakes if desired, set aside
2. In a skillet over medium-high heat, add the oil
3. Once heated, add in the shallot and cook, stirring occasionally for 2 minutes, or until softened
4. Add in the ground chicken and then season generously with salt and pepper, sauté breaking up any lumps with a wooden spoon, and cook until almost golden brown, about 3 to 4 minutes
5. Add in the garlic and ginger, cook until aromatic, about 1 minute
6. Add in the sauce and bring to a rapid simmer. Reduce the heat and simmer until the sauce is slightly thickened, about 4 minutes, taste and adjust the seasoning with salt and pepper
7. Divide the lettuce and quinoa between serving bowls and add the chicken
8. Top with shredded microgreens and sliced radishes
9. Garnish with sesame seeds and green onions
10. Enjoy!

Nutritional Facts Per Serving |Calories: 251 |Carbs: 27g |Total Fat: 10g |Protein: 14g

Butternut Squash Carbonara with Sage & Pancetta

If you like carbonara, then you'll love this Butternut Squash Noodle Carbonara! This healthy and comforting dish features crisp butternut squash noodles tossed in a cheesy, carbonara sauce and topped with pancetta and fresh sage.

Prep Time: 15 Minutes
Cook Time: 20 Minutes
Total Time: 35 Minutes
Yields: 4 Servings

Ingredients:

- 1 medium butternut squash, peeled, ends cut and spiralized, 1 lb. of noodles
- 2 whole large eggs plus 2 yolks
- 2 Tbsp. extra virgin olive oil, divided
- 4 oz. pancetta, diced or substitute with diced bacon
- 1 Tbsp. fresh sage, finely chopped, plus more for garnish
- 1/3 cup freshly grated pecorino romano, packed plus more for garnish
- 1/3 cup Parmesan, packed, freshly grated
- ½ yellow onion, finely chopped
- Vegetable Stock or Chicken Stock, optional
- Kosher Salt, to taste
- Ground Black Pepper, to taste

Directions:

1. Preheat oven to 400 degrees F
2. In a mixing bowl, prepare the carbonara sauce by whisking together the eggs, yolks, Parmesan and pecorino, then season with a pinch of salt and pepper. Whisk until the ingredients are well combined, set aside
3. In a large skillet over medium-high heat, add 2 Tbsp. of oil
4. Once heated, add in the pancetta and reduce heat to medium, cook, stirring occasionally, until crisp, about 5-7 minutes
5. Add in the sage and stir to combine, then use a slotted spoon to transfer the pancetta and sage to a small bowl, set aside
6. Add in the onion to the skillet and season generously with salt and pepper. Cook, stirring occasionally until the onion is translucent, about 4 to 5 minutes, then reduce the heat to low and add the pancetta and sage back into the skillet
7. In the meanwhile, bake the noodles by tossing the butternut squash noodles with 1 tbsp of the oil and season generously with salt and pepper
8. Bake for 10-15 minutes, or until the noodles are 'al dente', tossing halfway through cooking

9. Transfer the pasta to skillet with onion and pancetta, toss to combine and then remove from heat
10. Slowly pour the egg mixture over the noodles, stirring constantly and then mix until the eggs have formed a smooth, creamy sauce
11. Add in the stock, 1 Tbsp. at a time, if needed for creaminess, then taste and adjust the seasoning with salt and pepper
12. Garnished with additional pecorino and sage, if desired and enjoy!

Recipe Notes:

- Make the squash easier to peel by microwaving it. Just use a fork to pierce a few holes around the squash and microwave the squash for 45 seconds to 2 minutes. Allow it to cool and then you can peel it.

Nutritional Facts Per Serving |Calories: 252 |Carbs: 2g |Total Fat: 22g |Protein: 9g

Italian Zucchini Salad with Cherry Tomatoes and Turkey Pepperoni

Bright and made with the freshest ingredients, this Italian Zucchini Salad with Cherry Tomatoes and Turkey Pepperoni makes for a wonderful lunch or light dinner.

Prep Time: 15 Minutes
Total Time: 15 Minutes
Yields: 8-10 Servings

Ingredients:

Salad:

- 6 zucchini and/or yellow summer squash, spiralized
- 1 pint cherry tomatoes, halved
- 1 green bell pepper, finely chopped
- 1 red bell pepper, finely chopped
- ½ cup or 30 pieces turkey pepperoni, sliced in half
- 1 cup shredded mozzarella cheese
- ¼ cup finely chopped red onion
- 2 Tbsp. Salad Supreme seasoning

Dressing:

- 1 tsp. Italian seasoning
- 1/3 cup red wine vinegar
- 1 tsp. Dijon mustard
- 1 Tbsp. olive oil
- 1 clove garlic
- 1 Tbsp. honey

Directions:

1. In a large bowl, combine the zucchini noodles, bell peppers, tomatoes, pepperoni, cheese, onion, and salad seasoning, toss to combine, set aside
2. Prepare the dressing by combining the Italian seasoning, red wine vinegar, Dijon mustard, olive oil, garlic and honey in a blender, until smooth
3. Pour the dressing over the salad and toss to combine
4. Serve!

Nutritional Facts Per Serving (1 heaping cup)|Calories:122.9 |Carbs: 12g |Total Fat: 5.5g |Protein: 7.9g

Mediterranean Lamb Meatballs with Hummus and Cucumber Noodles

Tender Mediterranean lamb meatballs served with creamy hummus and fresh cucumber noodles, this dish is an easy meal you can make any day of the week!

Prep Time: 15 Minutes
Cook Time: 10 Minutes
Total Time: 25 Minutes
Yields: 6 Servings

Ingredients:

For the meatballs

- 1 lb. ground lamb
- ½ cup chopped white onion
- 3 garlic cloves, chopped
- 2 ½ tsp. dried oregano
- 1 tsp. ground cumin
- ½ tsp. coriander
- ½ tsp. red pepper flakes
- 1 tbsp. chopped fresh parsley
- Salt, to taste

Noodles:

- 1 English seedless cucumber
- 1 Tbsp. freshly squeezed lemon juice
- 2 Tbsp. extra virgin olive oil
- Salt, to taste
- Pepper, to taste
- 6 cups spinach (or arugula or other preferred green)
- 1 cup halved cherry tomatoes
- 1 ½ heaping cups hummus

Garnish:

- Feta, crumbled
- Dill, chopped

Directions:

1. Preheat the broiler
2. Line a baking sheet with parchment paper
3. In a food processor, combined the onion, garlic, and parsley, pulse until finely chopped
4. Transfer the mixture to a medium bowl and then add the lamb, oregano, cumin, coriander, red pepper flakes, and season with salt, mix until fully combined

5. With your clean hands, form 12 medium meatballs and set them on the prepared baking sheet
6. Broil for 8 to 10 meatballs, until they are browned on top but still slightly pink inside
7. In the meantime, spiralize the cucumbers to create the noodles and trim with kitchen shears
8. In a medium bowl, whisk together the lemon and olive oil, season with salt and pepper
9. Add in the spinach and tomatoes, toss well to combine and then set aside
10. Spread the hummus out on the plates and on each plate, top with the spinach salad, cucumber noodles, and then garnish with feta and dill
11. Serve!

Nutritional Facts Per Serving Size |Calories: 403 |Carbs: 14g |Total Fat:31g |Protein: 18g

Garlic Honey Ginger Chicken and Carrot Noodle Bowls

Sweet, savory and a little sticky, this healthy dish features a crispy baked chicken over crunchy spiralized carrot noodles that beats greasy take-out any day of the week.

Prep Time: 15 Minutes
Cook Time: 25 Minutes
Total Time: 40 Minutes
Yields: 4 Servings

Ingredients:

- 1 lb. boneless skinless chicken breasts, cut into bite sized pieces, about 1- 1 ½" cubes)
- 5-6 large carrots – peeled, ends trimmed and spiralized
- ½ cup cornstarch
- ½ tsp. salt, plus more to taste
- ¼ tsp. fresh cracked black pepper, plus more to taste
- ¼ cup and 1 Tbsp. vegetable oil or Canola, separated
- Crushed red pepper flakes, to taste

Sauce:

- 8 cloves garlic, minced
- 6 Tbsp. reduced sodium soy sauce
- ¼ cup sake
- ½ cup honey
- ¼ cup fresh ginger, grated
- 1/8 tsp. kosher salt

Garnish:

- ½ cup scallions, thinly sliced
- Sesame seeds, to taste

Directions:

1. Preheat oven to 400 degrees F
2. Prepare an 8x11 baking pan with cooking spray
3. Place the chicken pieces, cornstarch, salt and pepper into a plastic bag, shake the bag until the chicken is well coated with the cornstarch
4. In a large sauté pan over medium-high heat, add in 1/4 cup of oil.
5. Add in the chicken - be careful not to overcrowd, and sauté until lightly browned, turning to cook on all sides, about 2 to 3 minutes - The chicken will still be raw on the inside
6. Transfer the chicken to a prepared baking pan and then spray the top of chicken with cooking spray

7. Bake for 15 to 20 minutes, or until cooked through
8. In the meantime, wipe the pan of excess oil and place over medium high heat, once heated add 1 Tbsp. of oil to the pan, once heated add the carrot noodles and a pinch of red pepper flakes. Cook the noodles, stirring frequently, until softened, for about 5 minutes. Season to taste with salt and pepper, then place in a bowl and set aside
9. Add the garlic to the pan and sauté until fragrant, for about 30 seconds to 1 minute and then add in the remaining sauce ingredients – minced garlic, soy sauce, sake, honey, grated ginger and salt. Bring to a simmer, whisking occasionally. Then simmer for 3 to 5 minutes or until the sauce in thickened
10. Once the chicken is done cooking, add it to the sauté pan with the sauce, toss to coat
11. Serve chicken over carrot noodles, garnish with scallions, sesame seeds and additional red pepper flakes, if desired

Nutritional Facts Per Serving|Calories: 533 |Carbs: 64g |Total Fat: 18g |Protein: 27g

Cucumber Chicken Waldorf Salad

The classic flavors of a Waldorf Salad are all updated thanks to a healthy cashew-based dressing, chicken and cool cucumber noodles!

Prep Time: 15 Minutes
Cook Time: 15 Minutes
Total Time: 30 Minutes
Yields: 2 Servings

Ingredients:

- 1 English cucumber large, spiraled ribbons
- 1 apple red, large
- ¾ cup red grapes halved
- ½ cup celery chopped
- 1/2 bell pepper sliced thinly, I used yellow
- 2 Tbsp. sunflower seeds toasted
- ¼ cup parsley chopped, to garnish
- 2 Tbsp. walnuts raw
- 1 chicken breast
- Moroccan seasoning

Tahini Dill Dressing:

- 3 Tbsp. lemon juice
- 1 ½ Tbsp. red wine vinegar
- 2 Tbsp. tahini
- 1 Tbsp. olive oil
- 1 Tbsp. fresh dill or ½ tsp. dried dill
- Pinch sea salt optional

Directions:

1. Place a skillet over medium heat, drizzle with olive oil
2. Season the chicken breast with the Moroccan spice season, then add to skillet and cook for 10 to 15 minutes, or until no longer pink in the inside
3. Spiralize the cucumber and apple using the small noodle blade, place in a bowl
4. Top the cucumber and apple noodle with grapes, celery, peppers, walnuts and sunflower seeds
5. Chop the cooked chicken and place the it on top of the salad
6. Garnish with parsley.
7. Add the lemon juice, tahini, olive oil and fresh dill to a blender and a pinch of sea salt and blend until smooth and creamy, add more sea salt to taste
8. Serve salads with the dressing

Recipe Notes:

- *Nutrition facts assume you use the whole amount of dressing. Most typically use half of the dressing in a salad.

Nutritional Facts Per Serving |Calories: 535 |Carbs: 39g |Total Fat: 30g |Protein: 32g

Mediterranean Pork Chops with Vegetables

Flavorful and bright, this Mediterranean inspired dish features boneless pork chops served with spiralized vegetables makes for a delicious, weeknight meal!

Prep Time: 10 Minutes
Cook Time: 20 Minutes
Total Time: 30 Minutes
Yields: 4 Servings

Ingredients:

- 16 oz. (8) thin sliced center cut boneless pork chops
- ¾ tsp. Mediterranean seasoning
- 1 small (6 oz.) zucchini, ends trimmed off, spiralized
- 1 small (6 oz.) yellow squash, ends trimmed off, spiralized
- 1 cup halved grape tomatoes
- 1 Tbsp. extra virgin olive oil
- ¼ tsp. kosher salt
- Fresh cracked pepper
- ¼ tsp. oregano
- 3 garlic cloves, sliced thin
- Cooking spray

Toppings:

- ¼ cup of pitted and sliced Kalamata olives
- ¼ cup of feta cheese, crumbled
- Fresh juice from 1/2 large lemon
- 1 tsp. grated lemon rind

Directions:

1. Preheat oven to 450 degrees F
2. Spiralized the zucchini and yellow squash
3. Toss the tomatoes with ½ Tbsp. of the olive oil, 1/8 tsp. salt, pepper, and oregano
4. Then place the tomatoes, cut side up, on a baking sheet lightly sprayed with cooking spray, roast for 10 minutes
5. Add the sliced garlic and roast together for another 5 minutes
6. Transfer the roasted garlic and tomatoes to a work bowl and set aside.
7. Reduce oven to 200 degrees F
8. Place a large non-stick skillet over medium-high heat, add the remaining ½ Tbsp. of olive oil and the zucchini noodles with 1/8 tsp. salt and sauté until tender, for about 5 minutes
9. Add the sauté noodles to bowl with tomatoes and place in the warm oven

10. Season the pork chops with Montreal seasoning or seasoning salt of your choice, set aside
11. Working in two batches, spray the skillet with cooking spray and place it over medium-high heat, cook half of the pork chops for about 1 ½ to 2 minutes on each side, set aside on a plate
12. Remove the vegetables from the oven, place in a bowl and toss with Kalamata olives, juice of lemon and lemon rind
13. Serve the vegetables over the pork chops and top with Feta cheese.

Nutritional Facts Per Serving 2 chops, ¾ cup veggies |Calories: 230 |Carbs: 9g |Total Fat: 9g |Protein: 28g

BBQ Shredded Chicken and Squash Noodle Bowl with Avocado and Cilantro

Change dinnertime up with these amazing bowl BBQ shredded chicken and squash noodle bowls! They're made with flavorful squash noodles topped with shredded chicken, avocado mash and a touch of cilantro.

Prep Time: 20 Minutes
Cook Time: 20 Minutes
Total Time: 40 Minutes
Yields: 2 Servings

Ingredients:

For the chicken

- ½ lb. boneless skinless chicken breast
- ¼ cup favorite BBQ sauce

For the pasta:

- ½ Tbsp. extra virgin olive oil
- 1 garlic clove, minced
- 1 pinch red pepper flakes
- 2 medium yellow patty pan squashes, spiralized, noodles trimmed

For the avocado mash:

- 1 avocado, peeled, pitted, insides cubed and lightly mashed with a fork
- 1 Tbsp. chopped cilantro
- 1 Tbsp. freshly squeezed lime juice
- Salt, to taste

Directions:

1. Spiralized the squash, trim with a knife and set aside
2. Place the chicken breast into a medium saucepan and pour in enough water to cover
3. Place the chicken over medium heat, bring to a boil, and simmer until the thickest part of the breast meat is no longer pink, for 10 to 12 minutes
4. Transfer the chicken to a bowl and shred the chicken with two forks, then transfer the shredded chicken to a medium mixing bowl
5. Prepare the avocado mash by combining the avocado, chopped cilantro, lime juice, and salt to taste, mix together until avocado is chunky and smooth, set aside
6. In a small pot over medium heat, add in the BBQ sauce, cooking until heated through, about 2 minutes.
7. Pour the heated BBQ sauce into the bowl with the shredded chicken, stir until chicken is coated well with the sauce, set aside
8. Place a large skillet over medium-high heat, add in the olive oil

9. Once heated, add in the garlic and red pepper flakes and cook for 30 seconds or until fragrant
10. Then add in the squash noodles and cook for 2 to 3 minutes or until al dente, or cooked
11. Plate the squash noodles into two bowls and top with BBQ chicken and the avocado mash
12. Serve!

Nutritional Facts Per Serving |Calories: 339 |Carbs: 20 g |Total Fat:18 g |Protein:39 g

Zucchini Noodles with Simple Bolognese Sauce

Classic spaghetti just got a delicious update thanks to easy-to-make zucchini noodles and homemade Bolognese sauce!

Prep Time: 10 Minutes
Cook Time: 36 Minutes
Total Time: 46 Minutes
Yields: 6 Servings

Ingredients:

For the Zoodles:

- 6 medium zucchini, spiralized noodles
- 1-2 Tbsp. olive oil
- 1 clove garlic, minced

For the Bolognese Sauce:

- 1 Tbsp. olive oil
- 1 onion, chopped
- 1 stalk celery, chopped
- 3 cloves garlic, minced
- 1 lb. ground turkey or ground beef
- 1 (28 oz.) can crushed tomatoes
- 1 (6 oz.) can tomato paste
- 2 bay leaves
- Fresh basil, chopped as garnish
- ½ cup dry red wine
- 1 tsp. dried oregano
- 1 tsp. dried basil
- ½ tsp. salt
- ¼ tsp. black pepper

Directions:

1. Spiralize the zucchini, set aside on paper towels to soak up any excess water - Add a sprinkle of salt to help soak up the water
2. Place a large saucepan over medium-high heat, drizzle in the olive oil
3. Add in the onion, celery and garlic, sauté until fragrant, about 3 minutes
4. Add in ground turkey or beef, and cook until crumbled and brown, drain the excess liquid as necessary
5. Add remaining ingredients and bring to a boil then reduce heat and simmer for about 30 minutes

6. In the meantime prepare the zoodles by placing a large, clean skillet over medium-high heat, then drizzle in the olive oil
7. Add in the minced garlic and sauté until fragrant
8. Then add in zucchini noodles, cook for about 1 to 2 minutes until tender, season with salt if necessary
9. Top the zucchini noodles with the Bolognese sauce
10. Serve and enjoy!

Nutritional Facts Per Serving 1 zucchini and 1 ½ cups sauce |Calories: 239 |Carbs: 24.6g |Total Fat: 6.4g |Protein: 24.9g

Greek Chicken with Zucchini Noodles

This Greek Chicken Zucchini Noodles dish is the perfect easy, healthy weeknight dinner. It's made with just a few ingredients and full of flavor!

Prep Time: 10 Minutes
Cook Time: 20 Minutes
Total Time: 30 Minutes
Yields: 2 Servings

Ingredients:

- 2 Tbsp. olive oil
- 2 zucchini, spiralized noodles
- 1 lb. chicken breasts, cleaned, pounded, and cut into 1-inch cubes
- 1/3 cup Kalamata olives, halved
- 1/3 cup sun-dried tomatoes in olive oil
- 1 cup marinated artichoke hearts
- ½ tsp. pepper
- ½ tsp. dried oregano
- 1 tsp. dried thyme
- 1 tsp. dried thyme
- 1 Tbsp. lemon juice

Directions:

1. Spiralize the zucchini, set aside on paper towels to soak up any excess water - Add a sprinkle of salt to help soak up the water
2. Place a skillet over medium heat, add the olive oil
3. Once heated, add in the chicken, pepper, dried oregano and 1 tsp. dried thyme spices, sauté until brown on edges, about 15 minutes
4. Once the chicken is cooked, cut it into cubes and add in Kalamata olives, sun dried tomatoes and artichoke hearts, cook for an additional 2 to 3 minutes
5. Reduce the heat to low, add in a splash of lemon juice and the spiralized zucchini noodles to the skillet, toss and cook until the noodles start to soften, about 2 to 3 minutes
6. Once combined, plate and serve!

Nutritional Facts Per Serving |Calories: 575 |Carbs: 20g |Total Fat: 31g |Protein: 52g

Chicken and Zoodles with Creamy Parmesan and Sun-dried Tomato Sauce

You'll enjoy having this Italian inspired dish that features sun-dried tomatoes, garlic and parmesan cheese infused in a cream-based sauce over crispy, golden pan-fried chicken strips and healthy zoodles.

Prep Time: 10 Minutes
Cook Time: 25 Minutes
Total Time: 35 Minutes
Yields: 6 Servings

Ingredients:

- 1 Tbsp. butter
- 1 ½ lb. skinless chicken thigh fillets, cut into strips
- 2 large Zucchini or summer squash, spiralized
- 4 oz. fresh semi-dried tomato strips in oil, chopped
- 3.5 oz. jarred sun-dried tomatoes in oil, chopped
- 4 cloves garlic, peeled and crushed
- 1 ¼ cup thickened cream, reduced fat or full fat or half and half
- 1 cup shaved Parmesan cheese
- Salt, to taste
- Dried basil seasoning
- Red chilli flakes, optional

Directions:

1. Place a skillet over medium-high, add the butter
2. Once heated, add the chicken strips and sprinkle with salt. Pan fry the chicken until golden browned on both sides and cooked through
3. In the meantime, spiralize the zucchini, set aside on paper towels to soak up any excess water - Add a sprinkle of salt to help soak up the water
4. Once the chicken is cooked, add in the semi-dried and sun-dried tomatoes with 1 Tbsp. of the oil from the jar - optional for extra flavor
5. Add the garlic sauté until fragrant
6. Reduce the heat, add the cream and the Parmesan cheese, simmer while stirring until the cheese is melted through
7. Sprinkle with the salt, basil and red chilli flakes to taste
8. Stir in the zoodles and continue to simmer until the zoodles have softened, about 5 to 8 minutes
9. Serve

Recipe Notes:

- If you can't find any semi-dried tomato strips (which are usually in a deli area), replace them with an extra jar of sun-dried tomatoes.

Nutritional Facts Per Serving |Calories: 394 |Carbs: 9.2g |Total Fat: 22.6g |Protein: 35.6g

Korean BBQ Steak Bowls with Spicy Sesame Dressing

Korean BBQ steak over bell peppers, scallions, and greens wonton strips topped with a spicy sesame ginger dressing makes for an unforgettable lunch or quick and easy dinner!

Prep Time: 20 Minutes
Cook Time: 10 Minutes
Total Time: 30 Minutes
Yields: 4 Servings

Ingredients:

For the spicy sesame dressing:

- 2/3 cup low sodium soy sauce
- ¼ cup mirin
- 1 Tbsp. fresh minced or crushed ginger
- 1 Tbsp. toasted sesame oil
- 2-3 Tbsp. brown sugar
- 1-2 Tbsp. spicy chili paste
- 5 cloves garlic

For the bowls:

- 1 lb. top sirloin steak, cut into very thin pieces
- 2 bell peppers, red and yellow, spiralized
- 2 handfuls of spinach

Toppings:

- Wonton strips
- Scallions
- Sesame seeds

Directions:

1. Prepare the dressing by adding the soy sauce, mirin, minced ginger, toasted sesame oil, brown sugar, spicy chili paste and garlic cloves into a food processor, pulse until smooth
2. Place the steak in a bag and pour in enough dressing to coat the steak. Reserve the leftover dressing for the salad in the fridge
3. Spiralize the red and yellow bell peppers, set aside
4. Place a very heavy pan over high heat
5. Once heated, remove the steaks from the sauce, discard of the remaining sauce and add the steak to the pan with a little oil, if necessary
6. Allow the steak to cook for 1 to 2 minutes, until golden brown, flip if necessary

7. Remove the steaks from the pan and allow it to finish cooking on a plate. How long you cook the meat for is dependent on how well-done you want your steak, but just keep it mind that it cooks quickly because it's sliced very thin
8. Combine the spiralized bell peppers, spinach and steak into the bowls with enough dressing to coat
9. Garnish with the sesame seeds, wontons and scallions
10. Serve!

Nutritional Facts Per Serving (does not include wonton strips) |Calories: 250 |Carbs: 15.4g |Total Fat: 7.7g |Protein: 26.7g

Chicken Sausage with Broccoli and Parsnip Pasta

Chicken and broccoli go so well together, but you can make them even better by placing them on top of spiralized parsnip pasta!

Prep Time: 11 Minutes
Cook Time: 11 Minutes
Total Time: 21 Minutes
Yields: 3 Servings

Ingredients:

- 1 bunch broccoli rabe, stems trimmed
- 2 links spicy Chicken Italian Sausage, casings removed
- 2 parsnips, peeled and spiralized noodles, trimmed
- ½ tsp. dried oregano
- 2 cloves garlic, minced
- ¼ tsp. crushed red pepper flakes
- ½ cup low sodium chicken broth
- ½ cup grated Parmesan cheese
- Kosher salt, to taste
- Black pepper, to taste

Directions:

1. Chop the broccoli rabe into 1-inch pieces, set aside
2. Place a large skillet over medium heat
3. Once heated, add in the sausage and oregano and cook, occasionally breaking up with a wooden spoon 6 to 8 minutes, until browned, transfer to a plate
4. Add in the broccoli rabe and parsnip noodles to the skillet with the garlic and red pepper flakes
5. Add in the broth and cook until the noodles are al dente, about 5 minutes
6. Return the chicken sausage to the skillet, add the cheese and stir to combine
7. Serve!

Recipe Notes:

- If you don't like broccoli rabe since it's bitter, broccolini or broccoli would also work in its place.

Nutritional Facts Per Serving (1 1/3 cups) |Calories: 265 |Carbs: 25g |Total Fat: 10g |Protein: 22g

Zucchini Lasagna Casserole

This healthy vegetable lasagna has all the flavors you love, plus it's made with yummy zucchini noodles, mushrooms and topped with mozzarella cheese!

Prep Time: 20 Minutes
Cook Time: 25 Minutes
Total Time: 45 Minutes
Yields: 6 Servings

Ingredients:

- 1 Tbsp. oil
- 1 lb. ground turkey
- 1 tsp. Italian seasoning
- ½ tsp. salt
- ¼ tsp. pepper
- 4 zucchini, peeled and spiralized noodles, trimmed
- 8 oz. mushrooms
- 1 jar marinara sauce (24 oz.)
- 1 cup ricotta cheese, divided
- 1 cup shredded mozzarella cheese

Directions:

1. Preheat the oven to 350 degrees F
2. Place a large skillet over medium heat, add the olive oil
3. Once heated, add in the turkey, Italian seasonings and cook until turkey is browned, set aside
4. Spiralize the zucchini into noodles, set aside
5. In a large skillet over medium heat, cook the zucchini, tossing occasionally, for a few minutes until softened
6. Transfer the cooked zucchini noodles to a plate lined with paper towels. Pat them down with more paper towels to absorb the excess moisture
7. Add the mushrooms to the skillet, cook until soften and then add them to the plate lined with the paper towels
8. Spray a large casserole dish with cooking spray and then layer the ingredients as followed: ½ cup marinara sauce, a portion of the ground turkey and mushrooms, a pile of zucchini noodles, and ⅓ cup ricotta cheese
9. Continue on layering two more times with the remaining ingredients and top with the remaining marinara sauce
10. Bake for 20 minutes, then remove from oven and sprinkle 1 cup of mozzarella cheese over the top and return to the oven for 5 minutes until the cheese has melted
11. Slice and serve!

Nutritional Facts Per Serving |Calories: 341.5 |Carbs: 23.9g |Total Fat: 15.5g |Protein: 28.7g

Seafood

Asian Salad topped with Salmon and a Ginger and Lime Dressing

This flavorful and bright Asian salad is made with salmon filets, fresh spiralized veggies and creamy avocado, all tossed in a lime vinaigrette!

Prep Time: 15 Minutes
Cook Time: 15 Minutes
Total Time: 20 Minutes
Yields: 4 Servings

Ingredients:

Salmon:

- 4 (5 oz.) salmon filets
- 2 Tbsp. soy sauce I use reduced sodium
- 2 Tbsp. olive oil
- Salt, sprinkle and then to taste
- Pepper, to taste

Salad:

- 8 cups mixed greens
- 2 carrots spiralized noodles, trimmed
- 1.5 cups cucumber, spiralized noodles, trimmed
- ½ cup cilantro leaves, loosely packed
- 2 Tbsp. candied ginger, finely chopped
- 2 avocados, sliced

Vinaigrette:

- 2 Tbsp. olive oil
- 2 Tbsp. rice vinegar
- 1 tsp. lime juice
- ¼ tsp. dijon mustard
- ½ Tbsp. brown sugar

Directions:

1. Preheat oven to 425 degrees F.
2. Prepare a large baking dish
3. Place the salmon in the baking dish and drizzle with the olive oil and soy sauce, sprinkle with salt and pepper
4. Bake for 12 or so minutes, until fillets are cooked through

5. Prepare the vinaigrette by adding the olive oil, rice vinegar, lime juice, Dijon mustard and brown sugar in a jar or bowl, shake or whisk to combine
6. Prepare the salad by adding the mixed greens, spiralized cucumber, spiralized carrots, cilantro, candied ginger and avocado slices to a large bowl, then divide the salad ingredients amongst 4 large bowls
7. Top with salmon, and drizzle with the vinaigrette.
8. Serve!

Nutritional Facts Per Serving |Calories: 425 |Carbs: 18g |Total Fat: 29g |Protein: 27g

Spicy Sesame Crusted Seared Tuna with Spiral Zucchini Salad

Ready in just 20 minutes, this salad features spicy sesame crusted tuna on top of a bed of spiralized zucchini noodles with an Asian inspired dressing!

Prep Time: 15 Minutes
Cook Time: 2 Minutes
Total Time: 17 Minutes
Yields: 4 Servings

Ingredients:

Seared Tuna

- 1 (8-10 oz.) Tuna Steak, or Ahi, Yellowfin or Sashimi
- 1 tsp. chili powder
- ½ tsp. ground coriander
- ¼ tsp. ground ginger
- 3 Tbsp. sesame seeds – mix of both black and white
- Olive oil
- Kosher salt
- Ground pepper, to taste

Salad:

- 3 large zucchinis, ends trimmed and spiralized noodles, trimmed
- 1 large carrot, julienned
- ½ small red onion, thinly sliced
- ¼ cup cilantro leaves
- 2 scallions, thinly sliced
- 1 red Thai chile, minced
- ¼ cup unsalted dry roasted peanuts, coarsely chopped

Dressing:

- 1 small lime, juiced about 2 Tbsp.
- 2 Tbsp. soy sauce
- 1 Tbsp. sesame oil, plus more for pan
- 1 Tbsp. vegetable oil
- 1 Tbsp. light brown sugar, packed
- 1 tsp. ginger, grated
- 1 clove garlic, minced
- ¼ tsp. crushed red pepper flakes

Optional Add-Ins and Garnishes:

- Micro Greens
- Shredded Red Cabbage

- Cucumber, sliced
- Avocado, sliced
- Spring Lettuce Mix
- Mango, sliced

Directions:

1. In a small bowl, whisk together the lime juice, soy sauce, sesame oil, vegetable oil, light brown sugar, grated ginger, minced garlic, crushed red pepper flakes, taste and adjust the seasoning with salt and pepper, set aside
2. Season the tuna steak on both sides with coriander, chili powder, ginger, salt and pepper
3. Place the sesame seeds on a plate and then add in the seasoned tuna, gently press to adhere the seeds and then turn to fully coat
4. Place a medium sauté pan over medium-high heat, drizzle in both the olive and sesame oil
5. Once heated, add the tuna and sear, about 30 seconds to 1 minute on each side depending on how well you would like it to be cooked - The sesame seeds should be slightly golden and the inside of the tuna should be rare
6. Transfer the tuna to a clean cutting board and allow it to rest for a minute, then cut the tuna into ¼" thick slices
7. Return the sauté pan to the stove, then add in the zucchini noodles and season with salt and pepper, cook for 3 minutes, or until the noodles are warm and al dente. Transfer to a bowl
8. Serve by adding the zucchini noodles, carrot, onion, greens, cilantro, scallions and Thai chile to a bowl, top with a drizzle of half the dressing and then toss to combine
9. Arrange the salad on plates and top with sliced tuna, sprinkle with peanuts
10. Serve with the remaining dressing on the side
11. Enjoy!

Nutritional Facts Per Serving |Calories: 225 |Carbs: 17g |Total Fat: 15g |Protein: 7g

Blackened Salmon with Garlic Zucchini Noodles

Wow your taste buds with this simple recipe for flaky Blackened Salmon with Garlic Zucchini Noodles!

Prep Time: 10 Minutes
Cook Time: 15 Minutes
Total Time: 25 Minutes
Yields: 4 Servings

Ingredients:

- 1.33 lbs. wild salmon fillets, skinless, if possible
- 2 zucchini, spiralized noodles, trimmed
- 1 cup cherry tomatoes
- 2 tsp. smoked paprika
- ½ tsp. salt
- ½ tsp. garlic powder
- ¼ tsp. pepper
- ¼ tsp. onion powder
- ¼ tsp. dried oregano
- 1/8 tsp. chili powder, more to taste
- 2 Tbsp. olive oil, divided
- 2 garlic cloves, minced
- 1 lemon

Directions:

1. In a bowl, mix together the salt, smoked paprika, garlic powder, pepper, onion powder, oregano, and chili powder
2. Using a paper towel, pat the salmon dry
3. Rub the spice mixture onto the salmon on both sides- If the salmon has skin, only coat the side with the fish
4. Use the spiralizer to prepare the zucchini noodles
5. Sprinkle the zucchini noodles with salt and place in a colander to remove any excess water
6. Place a heavy skillet over medium-high heat, drizzle in half the olive oil
7. Once heated, cook the salmon for 3 to 4 minutes per side, transfer from the pan and set aside, tent with foil to keep warm
8. Add in the remaining olive oil to the pan, and add the garlic, cook for 1 minute
9. Then add in the zucchini noodles and tomatoes, cook for 3 to 5 minutes until al dente, season with salt and pepper to taste
10. Serve the salmon on top of the zucchini noodles with lemon

Nutritional Facts Per Serving (6 oz. Salmon and 1 cup of Noodles)| Calories: 331 |Carbs: 10g |Total Fat: 17g |Protein: 36g

Grilled Lemon Butter Halibut with Zucchini Noodles

With spiralized zucchini noodles and a grilled lemon butter halibut, you'll thoroughly enjoy having this delicious dish for dinner.

Prep Time: 5 Minutes
Cook Time: 15 Minutes
Total Time: 20 Minutes
Yields: 2 Servings

Ingredients:

- 2 skinless halibut filets (6 oz.) Fresh, or frozen and thawed
- 3 medium zucchini, spiralized noodles, trimmed
- 2 large cloves garlic, peeled and minced
- 4 Tbsp. clarified butter, ghee or butter
- Juice of one small lemon
- ½ cup roasted pine nuts
- 3 Tbsp. chives
- 2 Tbsp. olive oil
- Sea salt, to taste
- Pepper, to taste

Directions:

1. Wipe down the grill with coconut oil, then turn on high heat
2. Place the halibut filets on a plate and pat them down with a paper towel to absorb any extra liquid
3. Season generously with the sea salt and freshly ground pepper.
4. Once the grill reaches 425 degrees F, turn the heat down to medium, and add fish, then close lid. Cook the fish for three minutes, then turn it, cook for two more minutes and remove from grill, set aside and cover with foil to keep warm
5. Spiralize the zucchini into noodles, set aside
6. Place a skillet over medium-high heat, add the butter, olive oil, garlic and lemon juice, sauté for two minutes
7. Pour half of the sauce into a small bowl, reserve it for later
8. Add zucchini noodles to the pan and toss in butter garlic sauce - If zucchini are a little dry, add a bit more olive oil - and add in 1/2 of the chives, toss, cook for 3 to 4 minutes, occasionally tossing, make sure not to overcook the zoodles or they'll get mushy
9. Sprinkle with the sea salt, pepper and pine nuts, toss.
10. Place the zoodles on plate, top with the fish, and spoon the reserved garlic butter sauce over fish
11. Garnish with the remaining chives and serve!

Nutritional Facts Per Serving |Calories: 326 |Carbs: 4.96g |Total Fat: 30.48g |Protein: 10.98g

Parmesan Crusted Shrimp with Italian Zoodles

Baked Shrimp Parmesan over Zucchini Noodles – it's a super easy, very light and delicious shrimp dish that's ready in under 30 minutes!

Prep Time: 10 Minutes
Cook Time: 20 Minutes
Total Time: 30 Minutes
Yields: 2 Servings

Ingredients:

For the Shrimp:

- 8 oz. peeled and deveined jumbo shrimp
- 1 large egg, beaten
- 3 Tbsp. whole wheat Italian seasoned breadcrumbs
- 1 Tbsp. panko crumbs
- 1 Tbsp. grated parmesan cheese
- Olive oil cooking spray
- Fresh black pepper, to taste

For the Zoodles:

- 1 tsp. olive oil
- 2 cloves garlic, crushed
- 1 ¼ cups crushed tomatoes
- Kosher salt
- Pepper, to taste
- 2 medium zucchini (14 oz. total), spiralized noodles, trimmed
- 1 oz. shredded mozzarella cheese

Directions:

1. Preheat the oven to 450 degrees F and spray a baking sheet with cooking spray
2. In a bowl, beat the egg, set aside
3. In a separate bowl, add in the breadcrumbs, panko and Parmesan cheese
4. Wash and dry the shrimp with paper towels, then season the shrimp lightly with black pepper
5. Place a few shrimps at a time into the bowl with the beaten egg to coat, then coat with the breadcrumb mixture
6. Then place the breaded shrimp on a baking sheet and spray the top of the shrimp generously with oil, then bake for about 6 to 7 minutes, turn the shrimp, cook another 3 minutes or until cooked through
7. In the meantime, use a spiralizer to create the zucchini noodles
8. Place a large skillet over medium heat, add the oil

9. Once heated, add the garlic and cook until browned, for about 2 minutes, then add in the crushed tomatoes, salt and pepper and simmer on low for 5 to 6 minutes
10. Once the shrimp is done, add the zucchini noodles and cook 1 1/2 to 2 minutes, stirring to combine with sauce
11. Place the cooked shrimp over the zucchini noodles, top with cheese and place it under the broiler for 1 minute, until the cheese melts
12. Serve!

Nutritional Facts Per Serving (5 shrimps and ½ of the zoodles)|Calories:375 |Carbs: 27g |Total Fat: 13g |Protein: 37g

Spicy Lemon Garlic Shrimp with Zucchini Noodles

Have something more than just a sandwich for lunch like this spicy shrimp with garlic, zucchini noodles and tomatoes, topped with a squeeze of lemon!

Prep Time: 15 Minutes
Cook Time: 5 Minutes
Total Time: 20 Minutes
Yields: 2 Servings

Ingredients:

- 1 ½ tsp. olive oil
- 4 oz. shrimp, peeled and deveined
- 2 cloves garlic, sliced thin and deveined
- 1 medium (7 oz.) zucchini, spiralized
- ¼ cup halved grape tomatoes
- ¼ lemon juice
- Pinch crushed red pepper flakes
- Pinch salt
- Fresh black pepper

Directions:

1. Use the spiralizer, create the zucchini noodles, set aside
2. Place a medium nonstick skillet over medium-high heat, add 1 tsp. of oil and crushed red pepper flakes
3. Once heated, add in the shrimp and season with pinch salt and pepper, cook for 2 to 3 minutes
4. Add in half of the minced garlic, continue to cook for 1 more minute, or until the shrimp is completely cooked through and opaque, then set aside
5. Add the remaining ½ tsp. oil and garlic to the pan, cook for 30 seconds
6. Then add in the zucchini noodles and cook 1 1/2 minutes.
7. Add the shrimp and tomatoes into the pan and squeeze the lemon over the dish, remove from heat
8. Serve!

Nutritional Facts Per Serving |Calories: 235.5 |Carbs: 14.5g |Total Fat: 9g |Protein: 25g

Cucumber Noodle Salad with Tuna

Transform a can of tuna into a healthy meal for lunch with this simple recipe for cucumber noodle salad!

Prep Time: 15 Minutes
Cook Time: 15 Minutes
Total Time: 30 Minutes
Yields: 3-4 Servings

Ingredients:

- 1 seedless cucumber, spiralized noodles, trimmed
- 2 ½ cups seeded and diced tomato
- 7 oz. canned tuna in water, drained
- 1.25 cup diced red onion
- 1 tsp. ground cumin
- ¼ cup olive oil
- 3 Tbsp. fresh lemon juice
- Salt, to taste
- Pepper, to taste

Directions:

1. Use the spiralizer to create the cucumber noodles and then pat the noodles dry, transfer to a large mixing bowl
2. Add the tomato, tuna, onion, cumin, oil, lemon juice to the bowl, lightly toss
3. Season thoroughly with salt and pepper, to taste
4. Toss again to combine, making sure all the ingredients are coated in the oil and lemon juice
5. Serve!

Nutritional Facts Per Serving |Calories: 310 |Carbs: 20 g |Total Fat: 19 g |Protein:18 g

Moroccan Salmon Foil Packets with Carrot Noodles & Chickpeas

Just season your salmon and create the noodles, and you'll be enjoying a delicious, flavorful meal in under 30 minutes!

Prep Time: 5 Minutes
Cook Time: 20 Minutes
Total Time: 25 Minutes
Yields: 4 Servings

Ingredients:

- 4 (6 oz.) salmon fillets, fresh or frozen, thawed
- 2 large carrots, peeled and spiralized
- Salt, to taste
- Pepper, to taste

Optional toppings:

- 1-2 Tbsp. chopped cilantro

For the Chickpeas:

- 1 (14.5 oz.) can chickpeas, drained and rinsed
- 1 tsp. olive oil
- ½ tsp. sea salt
- ½ tsp. cumin
- ½ tsp. smoked paprika

For the Sauce:

- 3 Tbsp. harissa, mild or spicy
- 1 Tbsp. olive oil
- 1 Tbsp. fresh lemon juice
- 1 ½ tsp. fresh ginger, grated
- 3 cloves garlic, minced
- 1 tsp. smoked paprika
- 1 Tbsp. honey

Directions:

1. Preheat the oven to 400 degrees F
2. Spiralize the carrots into noodles and toss chickpeas with olive oil, cumin, sea salt, and smoked paprika until thoroughly coated
3. Cut heavy duty foil into four pieces (about 18x12 in. each), evenly divide the carrot noodles and chickpeas in the center of each piece
4. Season the salmon fillets with salt and pepper, place it skin side down on top of the carrot noodles and chickpeas, to make four foil packets

5. In a small bowl, combine the harissa, olive oil, lemon juice, ginger, honey, garlic and smoked paprika, whisk until combined, then spoon the sauce over the top of each salmon fillet
6. Make the packets by folding the sides of the foil together to seal, making sure to cover the fish completely
7. Place the foil packets on a large baking sheet
8. Bake in the oven for about 20 minutes, or until salmon is cooked through
9. Unwrap the foil and top with chopped cilantro
10. Enjoy!

Nutritional Facts Per Serving 1 Foil Packet |Calories: 469 |Carbs: 33.5g |Total Fat: 13.4g |Protein: 49.2g

Seared Tilapia with Spiralized Zucchini

You'll definitely have this recipe Seared Tilapia with Spiralized Zucchini in heavy rotation after making it just once! So what are you waiting for?

Prep Time: 5 Minutes
Cook Time: 20 Minutes
Total Time: 25 Minutes
Yields: 4 Servings

Ingredients:

- 4 (1 ½ lbs.) small tilapia fillets
- 1 ½ lbs. zucchini, spiralzed noodles, trimmed
- 1 Tbsp. capers
- 3 Tbsp. extra-virgin olive oil
- 1 lemon, thinly sliced
- 2 cloves garlic, thinly sliced
- ½ cup fresh flat-leaf parsley, chopped
- Kosher salt, to taste
- Freshly ground black pepper, to taste

Directions:

1. Preheat oven to 475 degrees F
2. Line a large rimmed baking sheet with nonstick foil
3. Spiralize the zucchini into thin ribbons
4. Transfer the zucchini noodles to prepared baking sheet, toss with 1 Tbsp. oil and ¼ tsp. each salt and pepper
5. Roast for 15 minutes, increase heat to broil and then continue to cook until golden brown, for 3 to 4 minutes.
6. In the meantime, heat 1 Tbsp. oil in a large cast-iron skillet over medium-high heat
7. Season the tilapia with 1⁄4 tsp. each salt and pepper, cook until opaque throughout, 2 to 3 minutes per side and then transfer to the plates
8. Add the remaining 1 Tbsp. oil to the skillet, then add in the lemon, garlic, and capers, cook, stirring occasionally, until the garlic is golden brown and tender, then toss in the parsley
9. Spoon the sauce over tilapia and serve with zucchini
10. Enjoy!

Nutritional Facts Per Serving |Calories: 289 |Carbs: 7g |Total Fat: 13.5g |Protein: 36g

Spicy Tuna Spiralized Vegetables Salad

Ready in just 10 minutes, this Garlic Chili Tuna Spiralized Spring Vegetables Salad makes for a flavorful lunch or light dinner!

Prep Time: 10 Minutes
Total Time: 10 Minutes
Yields: 2 Servings

Ingredients:

- 5 oz. wild caught canned tuna, drained
- 3 sweet baby spring turnips or 2 regular turnips, spiralized noodles
- 1-2 cucumbers, spiralized
- 1 tsp. minced garlic, about 3 cloves
- ¼ - 1/3 cup chopped shallot or red onion
- 1 small chili red pepper or cayenne pepper, sliced
- 2-3 Tbsp. olive oil, with a pinch of ground chili pepper mixed in it
- ¼ cup mayo
- 1 tsp. mustard powder
- Salt, to taste
- Pepper, to taste

Garnish:

- Cilantro
- Red pepper flakes or a pinch of cayenne to top

Directions:

1. Spiralize the turnips and cucumbers into noodles
2. Place the noodles in a bowl together with a pinch of salt and cover, then place it in the fridge while you prepare the sauce
3. In another bowl, mix together the mayo, mustard powder, lemon juice, garlic, onion, salt and pepper to taste, set aside
4. Drain the tuna, place it into a bowl and separate the tuna into pieces, mix in the olive oil and a pinch of chili pepper
5. Remove the spiralized cucumber and turnip noodles from fridge, drain any excess water from the bowl and gently pat the vegetables dry with a towel - Repeat until the water is removed
6. In a bowl, add in the spiralized vegetables, mix in mayo mixture, then add in the tuna and chili red pepper, mix again
7. Drizzle in olive oil and a few sprinkles of chili pepper on top, if desired
8. Garnish with the cilantro, extra lemon, salt and pepper
9. Serve!

Recipe Note:

- If you don't like mayonnaise, feel free to use Greek yogurt or sour cream. Also, you can refrigerate leftovers in the fridge for up to 3 days.

Nutritional Facts Per Serving ½ recipe |Calories: 302 |Carbs: 9.6g |Total Fat: 23.9g |Protein: 14.5g

Sweets

Baked Spiralized Apple Chips

Spiralized cinnamon and sugar apple chips are super easy and crisp baked treat that's also really healthy.

Prep Time: 10 Minutes
Cook Time: 2 Hours
Total Time: 2 Hours 10 Minutes
Yields: 3 Servings

Ingredients:

- 2 apples, Gala
- 2 tsp. granulated sugar
- 1 tsp. ground cinnamon

Directions:

1. Preheat oven to 250 degrees F
2. Line a baking sheet or two with parchment paper, set aside
3. Spiralize the apples using the large core slicing blade - Making the apple slice are the same thickness, cut into one half of the spiralized apple using a paring knife to help separate the apple slices into singular rings
4. Place the slices into a bowl
5. In a separate small bowl, mix together the sugar and cinnamon
6. Sprinkle the cinnamon and sugar mixture over the spiralized apple slices, gently toss them in the bowl to ensure they're evenly coated
7. Arrange the slices in a single layer with a little bit of space between them on the prepared baking sheet
8. Bake the apple slices for one hour, and then flip each apple slice over
9. Once flipped, bake the apples slices for another hour, and then shut the oven off
10. Allow the apple chips sit in the oven until mostly cooled to crisps them up
11. Enjoy!

Recipe Notes

- You can store the apples in airtight container for several days.

Nutritional Facts Per Serving |Calories: 65 |Carbs: 18g

Carrot Cake Muffins with Coconut Cream Frosting

If you're a fan of carrot cake, then you'll just love these soft carrot cake muffins topped with coconut cream frosting.

Prep Time: 15 Minutes
Cook Time: 25 Minutes
Total Time: 40 Minutes
Yields: 12 Muffins

Ingredients:

For the muffins:

- 1 large carrot, sprialized noodle, chopped
- 4 eggs
- 8 pitted dried dates, finely chopped
- ¼ cup coconut oil
- 1 tsp. vanilla extract
- ½ cup coconut flour
- 1 tsp. baking powder
- 2 tsp. cinnamon
- ½ tsp. nutmeg
- Pinch of salt
- Lightly chopped pecans, to garnish

For the frosting:

- 1 (14.5 oz.) can full-fat coconut milk, refrigerated overnight
- 1 tsp. vanilla extract
- 1 Tbsp. maple syrup

Directions:

1. Preheat oven to 350 degrees F and grease a 12-cup muffin pan
2. Using the spiralizer to create the carrot noodles, chop
3. Add the dates and coconut oil to the food processor and process until smooth
4. Transfer the date mixture to a large mixing bowl and add in the eggs and vanilla, beat the mixture until well combined
5. Add in the coconut flour, cinnamon, salt and baking powder, stir until combined
6. Fold in the spiralized carrots and mix to combine
7. Fill the greased muffin tin with the batter
8. Bake for 25 to 28 minutes or until an inserted toothpick comes out clean
9. Allow the muffins to cool for 5 to 10 minutes
10. While the muffins cool, prepare the cream frosting

11. Scoop all of the solids off the top of the coconut milk can, place it into a stand mixer or medium mixing bowl, along with the vanilla and maple syrup, beat until the frosting has peaks
12. Frost the muffins and serve!

Nutritional Facts Per Serving (1 muffin) |Calories: 181 |Carbs: 21g |Total Fat: 13g |Protein: 3g

Almond Butter Apple Bark with Coconut Flakes and Sea Salt

Make the best apple bark you've ever tasted with this amazing recipe Almond Butter Apple Bark with crispy Coconut Flakes and a pinch of Sea Salt.

Prep Time: 10 Minutes
Cook Time: 1 Hour
Total Time: 1 Hour 10 Minutes
Yields: 24 Bark Bars

Ingredients:

- 10 oz. bag chocolate chips
- 2 medium honeycrisp apples, spiraized noodles, trimmed
- 1 ½ Tbsp. almond butter
- 3 tsp. coconut flakes
- 2 Tbsp. sliced almonds
- Sea salt, to sprinkle, about 1 tsp.

Directions:

1. Line a 17" x 11" baking sheet with parchment paper, set aside.
2. Place a non-stick pot over medium heat, add the chocolate to melt while stirring it slowly
3. Transfer the chocolate to a large bowl, add in the apple noodles and stir well until the apple noodles break up and it's well combined with the chocolate
4. Pour the chocolate-apple mixture on to the prepared baking sheet in one even thin layer
5. Top it evenly with almond butter by the 1/2 teaspoon, coconut flakes and almonds
6. Sprinkle lightly with sea salt
7. Transfer the baking sheet to the freezer, chill for at least 1 hour or until hardened
8. Once done, cut the chocolate into 24 squares
9. Enjoy!

Recipe Note:

- If you don't have a non-stick pot, you can also boil water in a pot and then place a glass bowl on to with the chocolate. Stir slowly to melt the chocolate.

Coconut Plantain Rice Pudding

Get a taste of the tropics while you dig into a bowl of coconut plantain rice pudding!

Prep Time: 5 Minutes
Cook Time: 10 Minutes
Total Time: 15 Minutes
Yields: 1 Serving

Ingredients:

- 1 1/3 cup vanilla almond milk
- 1 medium-ripe plantain, peeled, spiralized noodles
- 1/8 tsp. cinnamon
- ¼ cup raisins
- 1-2 tsp. coconut flakes

Directions:

1. Spiralize the plantain into noodles
2. Then place the plantain noodles into a food processor, pulse until made into rice-like bits
3. Place plantain "rice" into a medium saucepan, add 1 cup of the almond milk and then bring to a boil
4. Once boiling, lower heat to a simmer and simmer for 10 minutes
5. After 5 minutes, the rice will start to reduce, once it has reduced (it will almost starts sticking to the bottom), add in the 1/3 cup of milk
6. Allow it to reduce, stirring occasionally until creamy.
7. Once done, remove from heat and add in the cinnamon, coconut flakes and raisins, stir until the cinnamon dissolves.
8. Pour into a bowl
9. Enjoy!

Nutritional Facts Per Serving |Calories: 242 |Carbs: 56 g | Total Fat: 5 g |Protein: 7 g

Pear Ribbons with Sweet Ricotta, Roasted Honey Walnuts and Fig

Transform simple pears into crisp ribbon that are topped with sweet ricotta, along with honey covered walnuts and figs.

Prep Time: 5 Minutes
Cook Time: 10 Minutes
Total Time: 15 Minutes
Yields: 2 Servings

Ingredients:

- 2 pears, peeled, spiralizer noodles, trimmed
- 6 black mission figs, halved
- ½ cup ricotta cheese
- 1/3 tsp. vanilla extract
- 1 Tbsp. honey
- ½ cup walnuts
- More honey to drizzle

Directions:

1. Preheat your oven to 375 degrees F and prepare two baking dishes by lining them with parchment paper
2. Use the spiralizer to create the pear ribbons, set aside
3. In one of these dishes, place the figs, sliced side up and dab them lightly with honey, using your fingers, bake in the oven for 10 minutes
4. In the other dish, add the walnuts and drizzle with honey and then mix to coat the walnuts evenly
5. Wait 3 minutes before the figs are done, then add in the walnuts
6. Once done, remove the figs and walnuts from parchment paper immediately, and set aside on a plate or in a bowl.
7. Prepare the ricotta whipped topping by pouring the ricotta cheese into a food processor and pulse until whipped, then place in a bowl with the vanilla extract and honey. Taste and add more vanilla or honey if desired
8. Arrange the pear ribbons on a plate, place some of the figs and walnuts around the ribbons and top with sweet ricotta and remaining walnuts and figs
9. Serve

Recipe Notes:

- This recipe calls for whole milk ricotta, but feel free to use part-skim to lower the calorie count

Nutritional Facts Per Serving |Calories: 296 |Carbs: 56 g |Total Fat: 21 g |Protein: 11g

Easy Spiralized Peach Pie Bars

Lovely peach filling and crunchy shortbread come together to create these yummy peach pie bars that everyone will love!

Prep Time: 15 Minutes
Cook Time: 45 Minutes
Total Time: 60 Minutes
Yields: 12 bars

Ingredients:

Shortbread Crust:

- ½ cup unsalted butter, melted
- ¼ cup granulated sugar
- 1 tsp. vanilla extract
- ¼ tsp. salt
- 1 cup all-purpose flour

Peach Filling:

- 4 small peaches
- 2 Tbsp. all-purpose flour
- 2 Tbsp. granulated sugar
- 1 tsp. ground cinnamon
- 1/8 tsp. ground nutmeg

Streusel:

- ½ cup old-fashioned oats
- 1/3 cup light or dark brown sugar
- ¼ tsp. ground cinnamon
- ¼ cup all-purpose flour
- ¼ cup unsalted butter, cold and cubed

Directions:

1. Preheat the oven to 300 degrees F and line an 8×8 baking dish with parchment paper and spray with non-stick spray
2. Prepare the crust by mixing together the melted butter, granulated sugar, vanilla extract and salt, in the order, together in a bowl. Then add in the flour and stir until well combined
3. Press the mixture evenly into the baking dish and bake for 15 minutes
4. In the meantime, prepare the peach filling by spiralizing each peach just until you hit the red part, and spiralize on each side of the peach.

5. Use a kitchen scissors or a knife to cut the peach noodles into small inch long pieces, then combine the peach pieces with the flour, granulated sugar, cinnamon and nutmeg in a large bowl until the peaches pieces are evenly coated, set aside
6. To make the streusel topping, whisk together the oats, brown sugar, cinnamon and flour together in a medium bowl
7. Cut in the chilled butter with a pastry blender or two knives until it's coarsely blended
8. Once the crust is done, remove it from the oven, and increase the oven temperature up to 350 degrees F
9. Spread the peach mixture around in an even layer on top of the warm crust - Making sure you press it down to fit tightly
10. Sprinkle the streusel on top and bake at 350 degrees for about 30 to 35 minutes or until the topping is golden brown
11. Serve!

Nutritional Facts Per Serving |Calories: 175 |Carbs: 92.84g |Total Fat: 9.99g |Protein: 2.87g

Pear Noodle Yogurt Parfaits

Opt for a healthy dessert with this parfait recipe that features pear noodles, Greek yogurt, plus the diced fruit of your choice!

Prep Time: 5 Minutes
Cook Time: 5 Minutes
Total Time: 10 Minutes
Yields: 3 Servings

Ingredients:

- ¾ cup diced fruit, bananas, blueberries or strawberries
- ½ cup Greek yogurt, vanilla, blueberry or strawberry
- 1 cup granola, favorite brand
- 2 medium pears, bosc or anjou

Directions:

1. Divide the diced fruit of your choice at the bottom of three mason jars
2. Top the fruit with ½ cup of Greek yogurt to each mason jar
3. Then top the greek yogurt with 1/3 cup of granola to each mason jar
4. Use the spiralizer to quickly create the pear noodles
5. Top the granola with pear noodles in each mason jar
6. Serve!

Nutritional Facts Per Serving |Calories: 137 |Carbs: 35.17 g |Total Fat: 0.13g |Protein: 0.73 g

Milton Keynes UK
Ingram Content Group UK Ltd.
UKHW050756250224
438379UK00011B/1245

9 781952 117039